easy reflexology

any age • any place • any time

Pauline Wills

Illustrated by
Juliet Percival

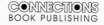
CONNECTIONS
BOOK PUBLISHING

A CONNECTIONS EDITION
This edition published in Great Britain in 2008 by
Connections Book Publishing Limited
St Chad's House, 148 King's Cross Road
London WC1X 9DH
www.connections-publishing.com

British Library Cataloguing-in-Publication data available on request.

ISBN 978-1-85906-265-4

3   5   7   9   10   8   6   4   2

The text in *Easy Reflexology* is from *The Reflexology Manual* by Pauline Wills, published by Connections Book Publishing (2004). The illustrations are based on photographs by Sue Atkinson.

Phototypeset in Meta using QuarkXPress on Apple Macintosh
Printed in China

Contents

Introduction   4

Pressure-point techniques   8

Massage techniques   12

STEP-BY-STEP TREATMENT   16

Giving a reflexology treatment   18

Reflex areas on the feet   21

Head and neck reflexes   28

Shoulder and chest reflexes   51

Abdomen reflexes   67

Lower body reflexes   96

Reflexes on the top of the foot   113

Finishing the treatment   121

ABOUT THE AUTHOR   128

Introduction

Originally known as reflex zone therapy, reflexology is a holistic healing method which involves pressure and massage of the reflex points found on the feet and hands. It is an extremely effective way of relieving stress, tension and fatigue and alleviating a wide range of aches, pains and common ailments, and is also highly beneficial used as a preventative measure to guard against ill health.

In the context of reflexology, the word 'reflex' is used in the sense of *reflection*, or mirror image. The feet (or hands) act as small 'mirrors' reflecting the whole organism. Reflexology teaches that a vital energy, or life force, circulates between the organs of the body, permeating every living cell and tissue. If this energy becomes blocked, the part of the body relating to the blockage is affected.

Energy blocks are reflected on the hands and feet in one or more of the energy zones located there. By using specific pressure techniques, blocks can be detected through the experience of pain, or through the presence of 'gritty areas', often referred to as crystal deposits. These occur in the part of the foot or hand that relates to the part of the body that is imbalanced. Reflexology uses pressure and massage techniques designed to dissipate energy blocks and break down crystalline structure. Through stimulation of the circulatory and lymphatic systems, and by encouraging the release of toxins, reflexology helps the body to heal itself.

HOW DOES REFLEXOLOGY WORK?

Ten separate energy currents – five in each half of the body – circulate between the head and the toes and the five fingers. These currents flow in longitudinal lines called zones. Within these zones lie all the organs and muscles of the body. The body is further divided into three transverse zones – at the level of the shoulder girdle (relating to the head and neck), the waist line (relating to the chest and abdomen) and the pelvic girdle (relating to the lower abdomen and pelvis) – and this allows for greater precision in locating the different reflexes (*see illustration overleaf*).

When the energy currents that flow through the longitudinal zones build up at certain points, they create an accumulation of energy – a blockage – at those points. These blockages interrupt the smooth flow of energy throughout the body, causing pain, disorder, disease or other problems which require healing. By removing these energy blocks, reflexology returns the body to a state of harmony, and allows the energy currents to flow freely once more.

Energy blocks in the zones can have many causes, both mental and physical: stress, bad diet, a lifestyle that is no longer beneficial, a broken marriage or relationship, for instance. The way to successfully remove the problem is to find the cause. The cause of a blockage may well be buried deep in the subconscious mind because the person finds it too painful to cope with. Alternatively, some people may be well aware of the cause but unwilling to discuss it, simply because they are not psychologically prepared to resolve it. Yet these energy blocks are obstacles which must be overcome. If the cause isn't found, a patient will continue to block the energy that the reflexologist has started to release. Equally, if the cause is known but the patient is unwilling to deal with it, the energy channels freed by the reflexologist will be blocked again by the patient.

Talk to the person you're treating, and listen to what they have to say. Try to uncover the root of the problem. If need be, suggest that they speak to a qualified counsellor. All methods of complementary medicine (of which reflexology is one) adopt this holistic approach: the patient is involved in the treatment, and is expected to take responsibility together with the therapist to effect a cure. (As the term implies, such therapies can work very well as a complement to allopathic medicine.)

HOW TO USE THIS BOOK

This book shows you – in easy steps – how to give a complete reflexology treatment through the feet. Divided into sections according to body reflexes, the treatment programme is easy to follow, and each step includes a quick-reference diagram highlighting the point or area of the foot being worked on, along with clear instructions on what to do.

First of all, you will need to practise the pressure-point and massage techniques set out overleaf (*see pages 8–15*). Once you have familiarized yourself with these, you can then begin treatment. Each section in the book includes relevant information on the anatomy and physiology of the body. In order to treat the body as a whole, you need to be familiar with the body's systems and organs – how they function both individually and in relation to each other – as well as with the various disorders associated with each. Always study the anatomy and physiology information in each section of the book first, before moving on to the step-by-step routine.

Once you have carried out the treatment a number of times, you may find that you no longer need to refer back to the book constantly for instruction. If this is the case, the wall chart shown on the inside of the book jacket provides a handy reference aid for the entire treatment routine, should you simply need a memory-jogger. The sections on the chart are colour-coded to match the book, so that you can easily turn to the relevant reflex section and step number, if you need to refer to the full instructions at any stage. Remember that you must always treat both feet when giving a reflexology treatment. Begin with the right foot, and complete the whole routine, before moving on to the left.

PLEASE NOTE: If you would like to practise reflexology professionally, you will need to obtain the necessary qualifications and insurance before you can treat members of the public. Check what qualifications are required where you live, and make sure any courses you attend meet recognized standards.

LONGITUDINAL AND TRANSVERSE ZONES

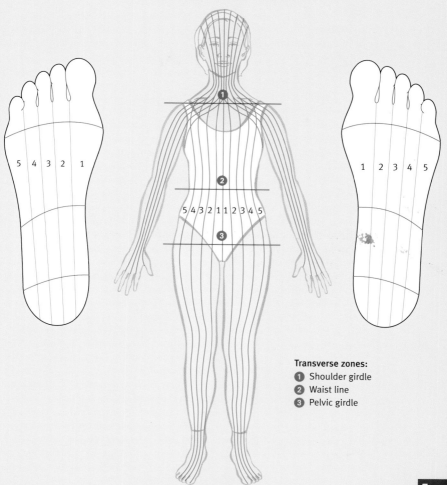

Transverse zones:

1. Shoulder girdle
2. Waist line
3. Pelvic girdle

Pressure-point techniques

Before attempting a full reflexology treatment, it is vital that you have mastered all the techniques you will be using, in order to feel confident that you're performing them correctly. Practise them first on your own hands – or feet, if you can reach them. There are five basic pressure-point techniques used in a comprehensive reflexology treatment. These are: thumb-walking, finger-walking, pivoting, sliding and pinching.

In general, the amount of pressure exerted when using any of these techniques should be adjusted to the person you're treating. You would use a firmer pressure on a healthy adult, for instance, than on a frail or elderly person, or a child. If you notice that the veins on the top or side of the foot are pronounced, use only very gentle pressure, to avoid the risk of causing a haematoma (bruise) – an accumulation of blood under the skin from vessels injured by a blow or disease.

Each technique is adapted to the particular reflex it is treating. Thumb-walking is used on the majority of the reflexes, with the exception of the very small points. As the name suggests, the thumb literally walks lightly over the surface of the skin. Finger-walking is a similar technique, but employs one or more of the fingers. Pivoting is used on small reflex points (for instance, the pituitary gland found in the centre of the big toe): the tip of the thumb is rotated slowly on the reflex.

The remaining two techniques are used less frequently, but can be useful for particular problems. Sliding, for example, can help break down crystal deposits. As the name suggests, it is performed by sliding the thumb over an area while maintaining a gentle pressure. It is used mostly on the soles of the feet, as it's a fairly robust action and can be painful on more delicate areas. The pinching technique is used only to treat lymph drainage, and simply involves pinching the relevant area using your thumb and finger.

THUMB-WALKING With the thumb bent, and only the outer edge of the tip of the thumb in contact with the foot, take tiny 'steps' all over the reflex being worked: press with the thumb, pull back to relieve the pressure (without losing contact), take a small step forward, press again, and so on. Keep the thumb bent, rather than constantly flexing and straightening it as it walks forward, as this could cause problems in the joint. Always position your thumb so that the flesh of the outer edge can fold in towards the nail, to prevent the nail being pressed into the foot. To begin with, you may find that your hands become very tired. This will improve as your muscles become stronger through practice.

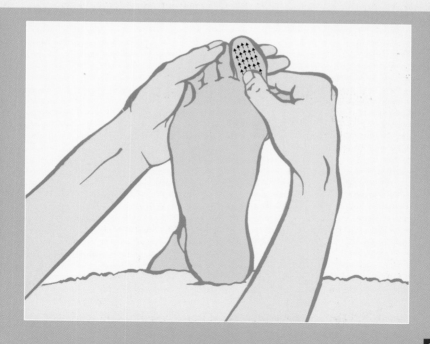

FINGER-WALKING This technique is applied mainly to the top and sides of the feet. Depending on which reflex is being worked, either one, two or all four fingers can be used. To treat the lymphatic system, for example, place the tips of all four fingers of your working hand on the top of the foot, close to the little toe, with your working thumb on the sole of the foot for support. Keeping your fingers bent throughout, gently press and pull back, walking all four fingers together down the top of the foot.

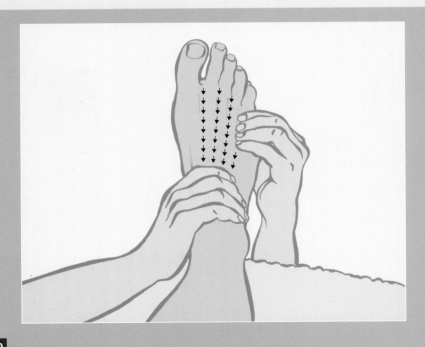

PIVOTING The position of the thumb and fingers is the same as for thumb-walking. Use the outer edge of the thumb, so that the skin overlaps the nail, as before. Press on the point you wish to treat and slowly and gently pivot on it, keeping your thumb in contact with the foot.

SLIDING Adopt the same thumb and finger positions as for thumb-walking. Press your working thumb gently into the foot and, maintaining the pressure, slide it along 1.25 cm (½ in). Pull your thumb back slightly before sliding along another 1.25 cm (½ in). Continue in this way until you have covered the reflex with which you are working.

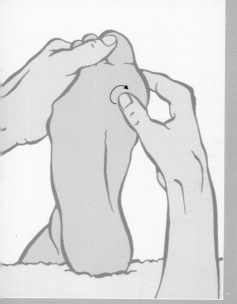

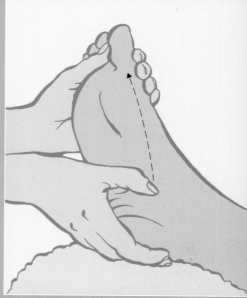

Massage techniques

Foot massage can be used both prior to treatment, to relax patients who are tense or under stress, and also after treatment has been completed, to stimulate energy. There are five basic techniques: wringing, kneading, stretching, finger-circling and stroking. These techniques are most effective when performed in this order.

Wringing helps to smooth out the feet by stretching the muscles. This is followed by kneading, which relaxes the person and stimulates body energy.

Stretching literally stretches the muscles, allowing the bones more freedom of movement. When performed on the feet, it makes the whole body feel as if it's being pulled upwards. It also helps to elongate feet that have been cramped up in tight shoes all day.

Finger-circling is a wonderfully relaxing technique. If your patient is very tense, try it before starting the actual treatment. Also, stroking can be a very soothing movement, ideal for removing tension.

Just as with the pressure-point techniques, adjust the pressure according to the person you are treating. To make sure your hands are quite smooth and dry, apply a small amount of talcum powder to them before massaging. You will find that they move over your patient's feet much more easily.

Again, it is useful to practise the techniques on yourself before you attempt to massage another person.

WRINGING Beginning at the top of the foot near the toes (*left*), wrap your hands around the sides of the foot, with the thumbs on the sole and the fingers on the top of the foot. Gently twist your hands back and forth in a wringing action (*right*) as you move down the foot towards the ankle. This is particularly beneficial for people who encase their feet in tight shoes, because the action of the hands stretches out the feet.

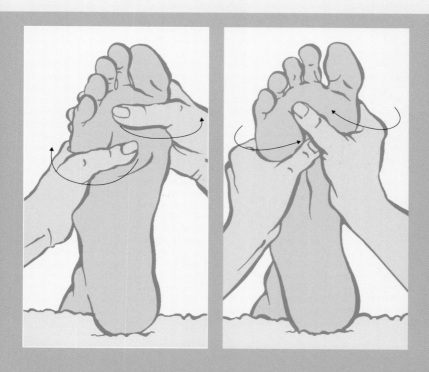

KNEADING Place one hand across the top of the foot and place the clenched fist of the other hand on the sole of the foot. Pressing both hands into the foot, make circular movements with both hands over the entire foot.

STRETCHING The position of the hands on the foot is the same as for the wringing action. Starting near the ankle, pull your hands up towards the toes. Repeat several times. The effect of this massage is to stretch the foot.

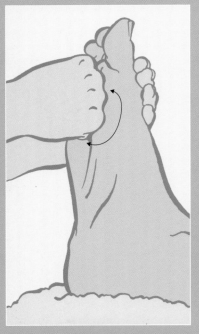

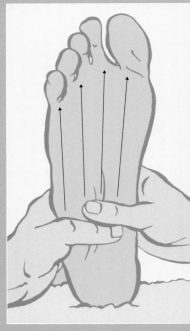

FINGER-CIRCLING Place the fingers of both your hands on the top of your patient's foot, and your thumbs on the sole for support. Keeping your fingers bent, gently make tiny circular movements with your fingers over the top and sides of the foot, and over the ankle bones.

STROKING Starting at the ankle, allow the fingers of both hands to gently stroke the top and sides of the foot in an upward movement towards the toes. This can be maintained for as long as you think it necessary.

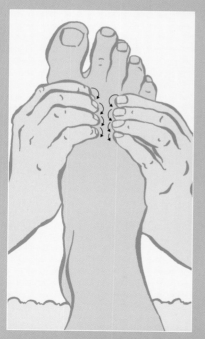

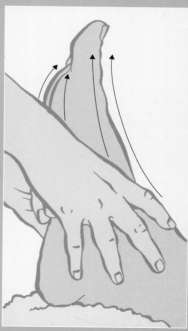

step-by-step treatment

You will now be guided, step by step, through a complete reflexology treatment. Remember to read the anatomy and physiology information at the beginning of each section first, before moving on to the step-by-step instructions. Also, don't forget that you must always treat the whole of the right foot before moving on to the left.

On the pages immediately following you will find advice on giving a reflexology treatment – where to do it, how long it takes, what to ask the patient, how to examine their feet – as well as detailed charts of the feet showing all the different reflex areas. Study these before moving on to the actual step-by-step routine. Familiarize yourself with the positions of the longitudinal zones, the transverse zones and the diaphragm. It will help you to locate the reflexes accurately. Some of them are only the size of a pinhead and may initially be difficult to find, but with practice you will soon learn to feel those points.

Finally, before you start a treatment, discuss what you intend to do with your patient. Holistic therapies treat the *cause* of the disease, not the symptom; and in order to find the cause you must encourage patients to talk. But remember the two golden rules: be a good listener, and never repeat anything said to you by your patient in confidence.

Giving a reflexology treatment

Ideally, a reflexology treatment should be given in comfortable and pleasant surroundings – a place that promotes peace and relaxation. This is important for both those giving and receiving treatment. Each treatment should last for about an hour (less on children, because they have smaller feet). There should be a minimum of three days between treatments; for most people, treatment is given at weekly intervals. This gives the body time to eliminate the toxins that reflexology has activated and to adjust to a new level of energy.

If you are giving someone their first treatment, they may not know what to expect and could be apprehensive. Explain what you're going to do before you do it. Make sure the patient is aware that they must tell you if pain is experienced on pressure, because this indicates a blockage of energy in

---

CAUTION

A few points to bear in mind before starting the treatment:

1 It is preferable not to give any treatment in the presence of certain disorders and conditions unless you are a fully qualified reflexologist. These include: osteoporosis, arthritis in the feet, heart conditions such as thrombosis and phlebitis, diabetes, and pregnancy – especially during the first sixteen weeks if there is a history of a miscarriage.
2 Similarly, treatment should not be given to cancer patients undergoing chemotherapy, radium or hormonal treatment unless you are a fully qualified reflexologist.
3 If you are in any doubt about giving a treatment, always seek professional advice before you start.

---

the part of the body relating to the reflex zone being worked. Also, give some warning of possible side effects, such as a feeling of tiredness, increased sweating and perhaps having to visit the lavatory more often, and explain that a condition can sometimes become worse before getting better. If patients are unaware of these factors, it can be very alarming if any of these side effects occur.

Always enquire into your patient's medical history, as this can provide insight into present problems. If the person you're treating is taking medication, on no account suggest that it be interrupted: certain drugs can produce severe withdrawal symptoms, and any suspension in the treatment programme could create problems for the person concerned. A patient's medication should only be stopped by the person who prescribed it.

If your patient complains of pains, or describes any other symptoms to you, be sure to ask if they have had it checked medically. If they haven't, suggest that they do so. Reflexologists are not allowed to make a medical diagnosis; even if you suspect that a person is suffering from a certain ailment, you can only describe it as an energy imbalance.

GETTING COMFORTABLE
After gleaning all the necessary information, seat the patient in a position that affords complete relaxation and also places the feet at a comfortable height for you to treat (NOTE: it is considered bad practice to support the patient's feet on your lap!). A reflexology treatment works towards an unrestricted flow of energy throughout the physical body. An uncomfortable seat or posture can create tension that impedes this energy flow.

The ideal position is one that allows the feet to be raised to a suitable height for treatment, the knees to be slightly bent to alleviate tension in the calf and thigh muscles, and the trunk of the body to be positioned at such an angle that the patient's face is visible to you: facial expressions impart important information.

A helpful hint: have a box of tissues handy. If someone has travelled a long way or has come straight from work, you may feel that their feet need washing. Never be embarrassed to ask someone to do this. In my experience, most people are only too happy to oblige!

OBSERVATION

Before starting the actual treatment, it's important to carry out a methodical observation of the feet, as they can supply valuable information. Start with the skeletal structure. Changes in this could indicate a disturbance in the energy flow within the reflex zone, resulting in a disorder in the corresponding part of the body. One example would be bunions – inflammation on the outside edge of the joint at the base of the big toe. These affect the reflex zones to the cervical spine and thyroid gland.

Look at the colour and state of the skin. Swelling in the feet could relate to congestion in the corresponding part of the body. If the swelling is around the ankle, it could indicate a kidney, heart or circulatory disorder. Another sign of heart and circulatory disorders is the presence of tiny pads around the base of the toes on the front of the left foot. Notice also the condition of the skin. If the skin is excessively dry, this could either be a sign of poor circulation in the outer extremities of the body, or it could refer to a hormonal imbalance. If the feet have been neglected and are covered in rough, hard skin, it would be expedient to suggest a visit to a chiropodist to have this removed.

Calluses and corns could point to problems in the body related to the zone that they cover. A corn on the outer side of the little toe, for example, could reflect an injury to the shoulder; a corn on the pad of one or more of the toes could mirror sinus problems. Finally, look at the nails. These can reveal a great deal about a person's health. If, for example, you find that the nail bed appears to be rather pale and you suspect anaemia, suggest a visit to a doctor.

Once you have completed your visual observations, you can then begin your reflexology treatment.

PRELIMINARY EXERCISES

You may find it helpful to do some loosening-up exercises with your patient first: rotation of the ankles and toes helps to alleviate stiffness in the joints and aids the release of any energy blocks.

Start with the right foot: place one hand underneath the heel to support it and, using your other hand, slowly and gently rotate the foot. When you have treated the ankle, move your supporting hand to the top of the foot, and use your other hand to slowly rotate each toe, holding each by its middle joint. Work in both a clockwise and anticlockwise direction, before moving on to the left foot.

Reflex areas on the feet

The charts on the following pages show the positions of all the reflexes on the feet, and the parts of the body to which they relate (*see pages 22–27*). Reflex areas are found on the sole, top, medial (inner) and lateral (outer) sides of both feet. Reflexes to the organs situated on the right side of the body are found on the right foot; those situated on the left side are found on the left foot. Note that some reflexes are located on one foot only: for example, the liver reflex lies on the right foot only, while the heart reflex lies on the left foot only. In addition, some organ reflexes are distributed across both feet.

Before starting your treatment, study these charts carefully to help you locate the reflexes accurately. For further guidance, the transverse and longitudinal zones are indicated, as well as the diaphragm (marked as a dotted line).

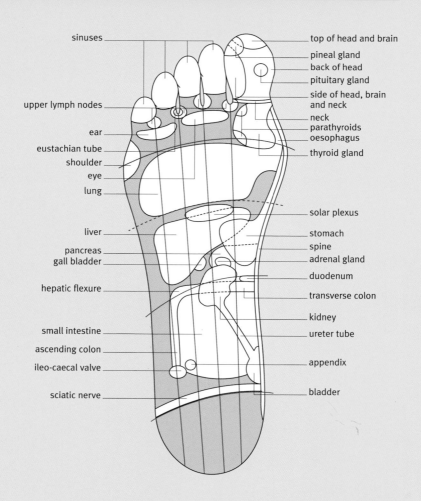

sinuses

top of head and brain

pineal gland

back of head

pituitary gland

side of head, brain and neck

upper lymph nodes

neck

parathyroids

ear

oesophagus

eustachian tube

thyroid gland

shoulder

eye

lung

solar plexus

liver

stomach

spine

pancreas

adrenal gland

gall bladder

duodenum

hepatic flexure

transverse colon

kidney

small intestine

ureter tube

ascending colon

ileo-caecal valve

appendix

sciatic nerve

bladder

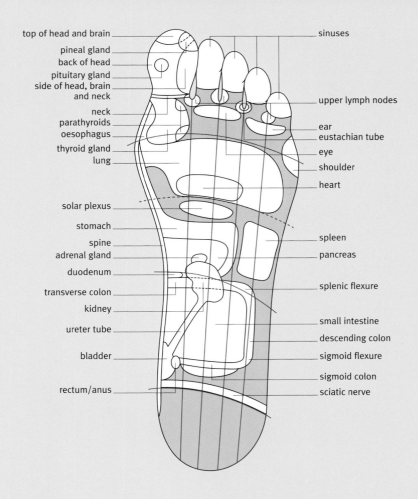

top of head and brain

pineal gland
back of head
pituitary gland
side of head, brain
and neck

neck
parathyroids
oesophagus
thyroid gland
lung

solar plexus

stomach

spine
adrenal gland

duodenum

transverse colon

kidney

ureter tube

bladder

rectum/anus

sinuses

upper lymph nodes

ear
eustachian tube
eye
shoulder

heart

spleen
pancreas

splenic flexure

small intestine
descending colon
sigmoid flexure

sigmoid colon
sciatic nerve

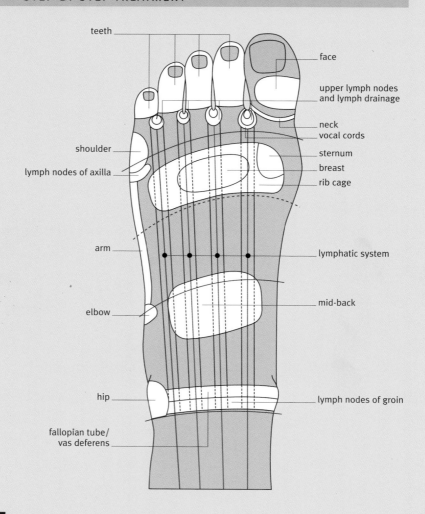

teeth

face

upper lymph nodes
and lymph drainage

neck
vocal cords

shoulder

sternum

lymph nodes of axilla

breast

rib cage

arm

lymphatic system

mid-back

elbow

hip

lymph nodes of groin

fallopian tube/
vas deferens

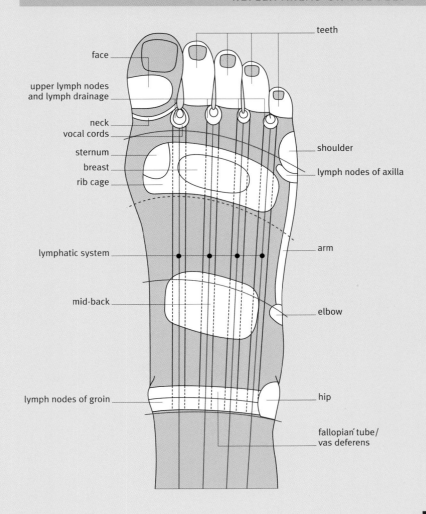

face

upper lymph nodes
and lymph drainage

neck
vocal cords

sternum
breast
rib cage

lymphatic system

mid-back

lymph nodes of groin

teeth

shoulder

lymph nodes of axilla

arm

elbow

hip

fallopian tube/
vas deferens

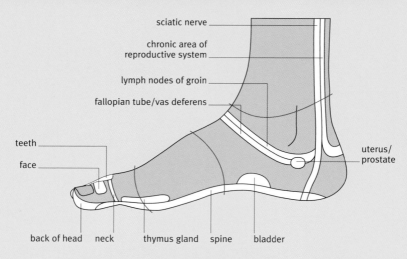

sciatic nerve

chronic area of
reproductive system

lymph nodes of groin

fallopian tube/vas deferens

teeth

face

uterus/
prostate

back of head   neck   thymus gland   spine   bladder

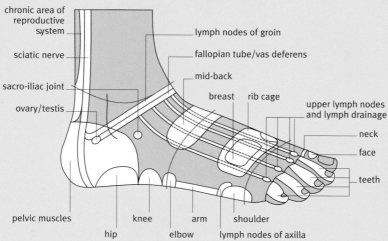

chronic area of
reproductive
system

lymph nodes of groin

sciatic nerve

fallopian tube/vas deferens

mid-back

sacro-iliac joint

breast   rib cage

ovary/testis

upper lymph nodes
and lymph drainage

neck

face

teeth

pelvic muscles   knee   arm   shoulder

hip   elbow   lymph nodes of axilla

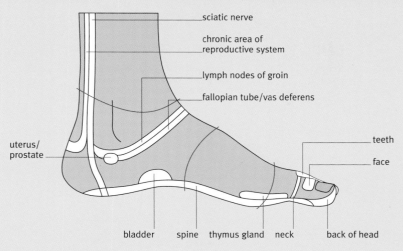

sciatic nerve

chronic area of reproductive system

lymph nodes of groin

fallopian tube/vas deferens

uterus/prostate

teeth

face

bladder spine thymus gland neck back of head

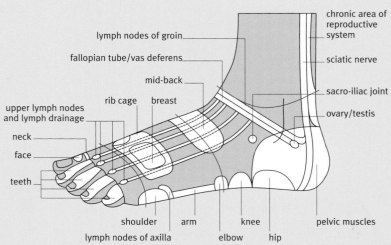

chronic area of reproductive system

lymph nodes of groin

sciatic nerve

fallopian tube/vas deferens

mid-back

sacro-iliac joint

rib cage breast

ovary/testis

upper lymph nodes and lymph drainage

neck

face

teeth

shoulder arm

lymph nodes of axilla

knee

elbow hip

pelvic muscles

Head and neck reflexes

The reflexes relating to the head and the neck are located on the five toes of both feet. Each big toe can be divided into five longitudinal zones corresponding to the head and brain area. All the head and neck reflexes are found in the first transverse zone, which covers the phalanges and ends at the metatarsals. Treatment should start with the pituitary gland and continue in the sequence given in the step-by-step guide. Working methodically in this way will ensure that none of the reflexes are overlooked. As you work the reflexes, take note of any that are painful. Return to these at the end of the session, so that you can give them extra treatment.

PITUITARY GLAND

This gland lies at the base of the brain, just above and behind the nasal cavity. It is only the size of a pea and is the master gland of the endocrine system. The pituitary gland consists of an anterior and a posterior lobe, each having different functions. The anterior lobe produces hormones which stimulate the thyroid and adrenal glands, affect sexual life and govern the secretion of breast milk. The posterior lobe secretes hormones that stimulate the muscles of the uterus during and after childbirth, stimulate the breasts to produce milk, cause the contraction of involuntary muscles and act as an antidiuretic. This reflex area is important for hormonal imbalances.

PINEAL GLAND

The pineal gland is approximately the same size as the pituitary gland and is situated just in front of the cerebellum, which lies low down at the back of the skull. Its principal function is to secrete melatonin, which affects the body's biological clock. If the level of this hormone in the blood is too high during daylight hours, it produces a condition known as seasonal affective disorder (or SAD). This gland also regulates the onset of puberty, induces sleep and influences our moods.

HEAD AND BRAIN
The head, containing the brain, controls and monitors all bodily functions. The brain is a soft jelly-like structure made up of about 1,000 billion neurons, and is one of the largest organs of the body. It is divided into four main parts: the diencephalon, the cerebrum, the cerebellum and the brain stem (which is a continuation of the spinal cord). The cerebellum is responsible for co-ordinating reflex actions and controlling posture, balance and

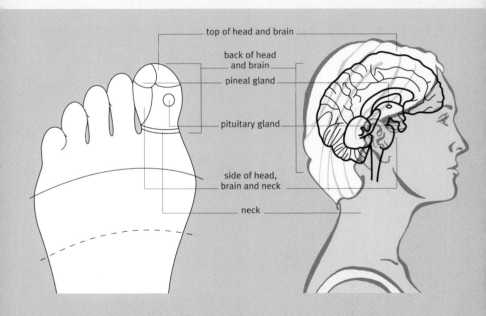

top of head and brain

back of head and brain

pineal gland

pituitary gland

side of head, brain and neck

neck

muscular activity. The cerebrum contains the nerve centres responsible for conscious thought and action. This reflex is important for conditions such as headaches, migraine, Parkinson's disease, epilepsy, cerebral palsy, multiple sclerosis, trigeminal neuralgia (or tic douloureux) and dyslexia.

VERTEBRAL COLUMN (SPINE)

The vertebral column is made up of thirty-three vertebrae. These are divided into seven cervical vertebrae (in the neck region), twelve thoracic (posterior to the thoracic cavity), five lumbar (in charge of supporting the lower back), five sacral, which are fused into one bone to form the sacrum, and four which are fused into either one or two bones to form the coccyx. The vertebral column encloses and protects the spinal cord, supports the head and serves as a point of attachment for the ribs and the muscles of the back. Treatment to this reflex is advised for back pain, and for diseases associated with the spinal nerves.

NECK

The reflex to the neck is found around the base of the big toe, a third of the way along the lateral border. Gentle rotation of the big toes can alleviate tension in the neck. If the toe joints are stiff, it may indicate rigidity in this area.

FACE

The reflex to the face, like the reflex to the back of the head, can be divided into five longitudinal zones. The right foot represents the right side of the face, and the left foot, the left side. All parts of the face, such as the eyes, nose, sinuses, teeth, lips and muscles, are included in this reflex. Problems related to the face, such as sinusitis, toothache, eye strain and Bell's palsy (facial paralysis), can be helped through this reflex.

VOCAL CORDS

The larynx is a complicated cartilaginous structure lying between the pharynx and the trachea. Running inside the larynx are two membranes

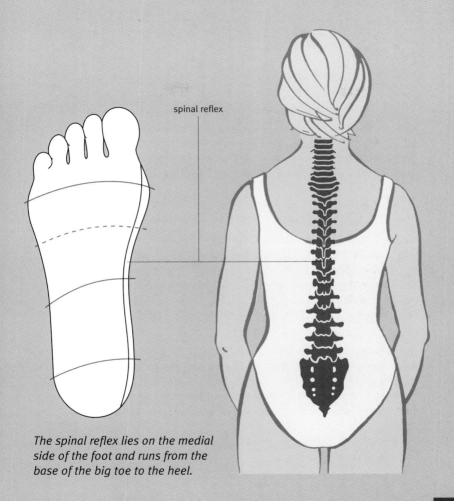

spinal reflex

The spinal reflex lies on the medial side of the foot and runs from the base of the big toe to the heel.

known as the vocal cords. Using these membranes for voice production is a highly complex operation of co-ordination between the breath, the lips, the tongue and the vocal cords. This is an important reflex in cases of laryngitis, pharyngitis and tracheitis.

SINUSES

The sinuses are cavities in the bones of the face and skull which are linked by narrow channels to the nose. They are situated in the forehead just above the eyes, in the cheekbones, and between and behind the eyes. The sinuses lighten the skull bones and serve as resonant sound chambers when we speak or sing. They are lined with a membrane that secretes mucus, which drains into the nose to be cleared. Inflammation of the sinuses can be caused by a viral infection, or a swelling of the mucous membranes associated with hay fever. These reflexes are important in the treatment of colds, catarrh and hay fever.

EYES

The eyes are the complicated and extremely efficient organs of vision. Set in their bony sockets, they are protected from injury. Self-focusing, self-lubricating and self-cleansing, they adapt to bright or dim light and to distant or near vision. This reflex is important for eye strain, conjunctivitis, cataract and all other conditions related to the eyes.

EAR AND EUSTACHIAN TUBE

Our hearing is one of the most sensitive and discriminating of senses. Sound is perceived by the brain. When sound waves fall on the eardrum, they cause it to vibrate. The vibrations reach the inner ear, causing the fluid in its cavity to vibrate in turn, thereby exciting nerve endings which carry the impulses to the brain. The eustachian tube starts at the back of the middle ear and opens into the throat. Its function is to equalize the pressure on either side of the eardrum. Both of these reflexes are important for conditions such as tinnitus, infections, deafness and vertigo.

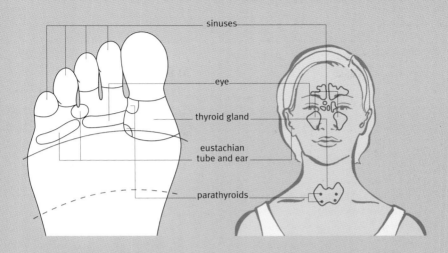

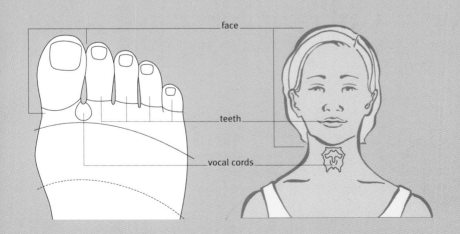

THYROID GLAND

The thyroid gland has two lobes which are situated on either side of the windpipe, just below the level of the larynx. These lobes are joined by a narrow strip of thyroid tissue. The thyroid is unique among endocrine glands in that it requires iodine to make one of its two hormones, thyroxine. Its hormones affect the metabolism of practically all the tissues of the body: they regulate the rate at which oxygen is consumed, are powerful growth promoters, and are necessary for the full development of the brain. Treatment of this reflex is important for cretinism, myxoedema, goiter and also imbalances in the reproductive glands.

PARATHYROID GLANDS

These tiny glands, usually four in number, are superficially embedded in the back and side surfaces of each lobe of the thyroid. The hormone secreted by these glands is called parathormone, and is concerned with keeping a steady level of calcium and phosphorus in the blood. The parathyroid reflexes are helpful for cases of arthritis, osteoporosis, muscle twitching and spasms.

TEETH

Every human has two sets of teeth. The first set of twenty primary teeth will usually have emerged by the age of three. By the age of twenty-five, the permanent set of thirty-two teeth have erupted. The reflexes for the teeth are important for conditions relating to dental problems, including abscesses, toothache and gingivitis – inflammation of the gums.

1   Starting with the patient's right foot, find the **pituitary gland** reflex in the centre of the fleshy pad of the big toe. Support the foot with your left hand and support the big toe with the fingers of your working hand. Press the reflex with the outer edge of your thumb, which should be slightly bent at the first joint. Make sure your nail isn't digging into the toe. Gently rotate on this point for a few seconds. This reflex can be very sensitive, so apply less pressure if your patient complains of pain.

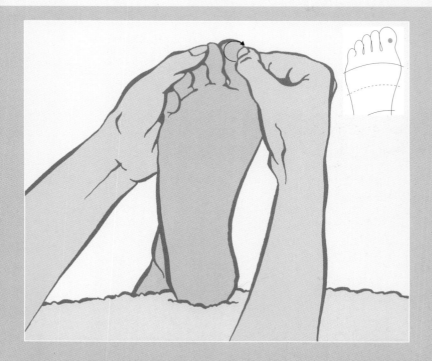

2 Move the starting position of your thumb to the inner side of the big toe, approximately 1.25 cm (½ in) down from the top. This is where the **pineal gland** reflex is located. Still supporting the foot with your left hand, approach this reflex with your working hand from above the foot. Use the fingers of your working hand to support the toe joint while you press the reflex with the outer edge of your bent thumb, and gently rotate on this point for a few seconds.

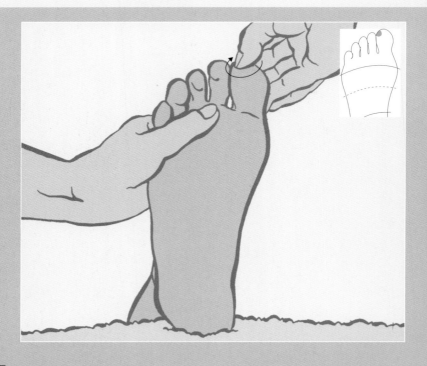

3 After treating the pineal gland, move your working thumb to the lateral side of the foot, at the base of the big toe. The reflex for the **back of the head** begins here, covering the whole of the fleshy pad on the toe. Support the foot with your left hand and the toe with the fingers of your working hand. Thumb-walk in six parallel lines from the base to the top of the toe.

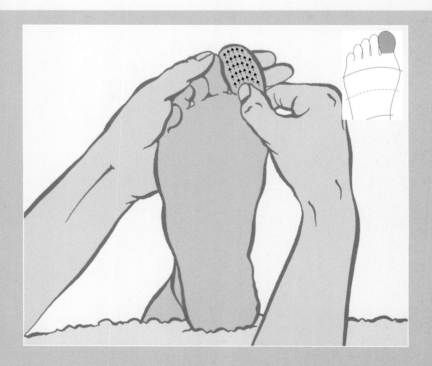

4   To work the area relating to the **sides of the neck and head** and the **top of the brain,** place your working thumb at the bottom of the lateral border of the big toe. Thumb-walk up the inside of the toe to the top of the toe. Change hands, using your other thumb to walk across the top of the toe.

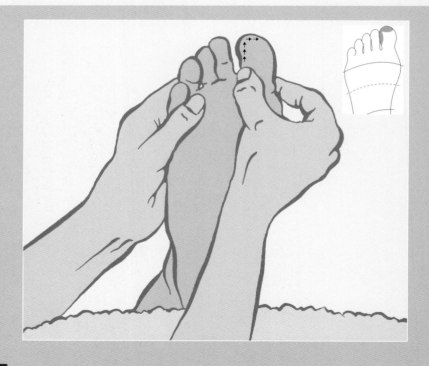

5 Keep your working thumb on the medial edge at the top of the big toe. Support the foot under the heel with your right hand, tilting it slightly to the left (*left*). Now thumb-walk down the **spinal** reflex, which lies on the medial border of the big toe and the medial side of the foot, just below the arch, to two-thirds of the way along the calcaneum (heel bone). When you reach this point (*right*), change hands and slide the outer edge of your right thumb back up the spinal reflex.

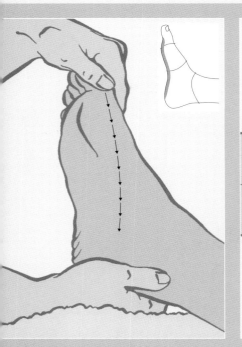
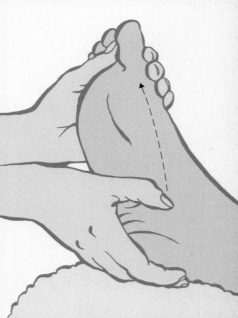

6 To treat the **neck** reflex, position your thumb on the outer edge of the big toe. Hold the front of the toes with your left hand and gently pull them back. Supporting the front of the big toe with your working-hand fingers, thumb-walk across the base of the toe.

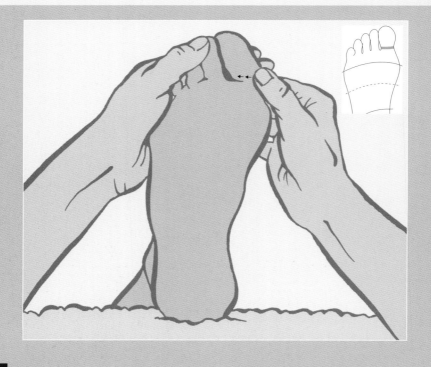

7   Without changing its position, use your working hand's first three
    fingers to walk across the **face** reflex found on the front of the big toe.
    Your working thumb should support the back of the toe. This area
    includes reflexes for the eyes, nose, teeth, lips and facial muscles.

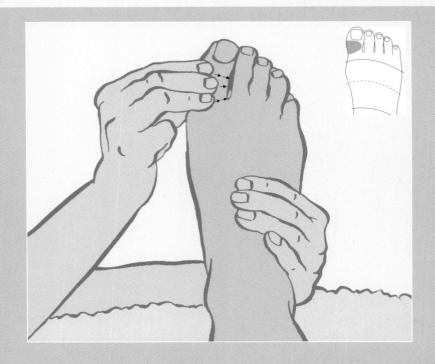

8   To treat the **vocal cords,** raise your working hand over the foot and place the index finger on the front of the foot between the big toe and the second toe. This is where you will find the reflex to the vocal cords. Place the thumb of your working hand on the sole of the foot, behind your index finger, for support. Using your finger, gently rotate over this area. This reflex is important for preventive treatment, as the larynx can become inflamed through excessive smoking or over-using the voice.

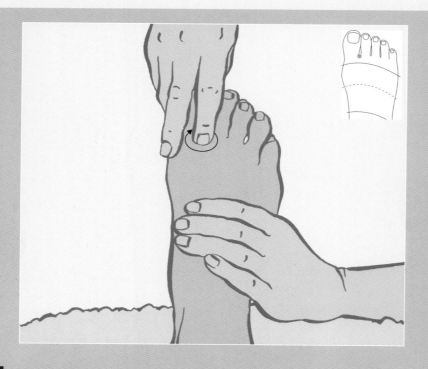

9   The back and sides of the four smaller toes contain the **sinus** reflexes. Support the front of the foot and gently extend the toes back. With your working fingers on the front of the toes, thumb-walk up the backs and sides of all four toes in turn, starting with the second toe.

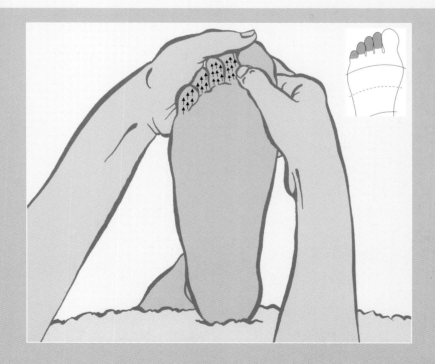

10   Keeping the toes extended back with your supporting hand, move
     your working thumb to the medial side at the base of the second
     toe. This is where the reflex area to the **eyes** is located. Thumb-walk
     across the base of the second and third toe.

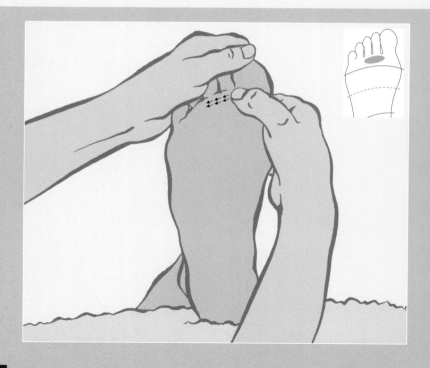

11 Thumb-walk along the base of the toes until you reach the web between the third and fourth toe. This is the **eustachian tube** reflex area. Gently rotate on this point with the outer edge of your thumb.

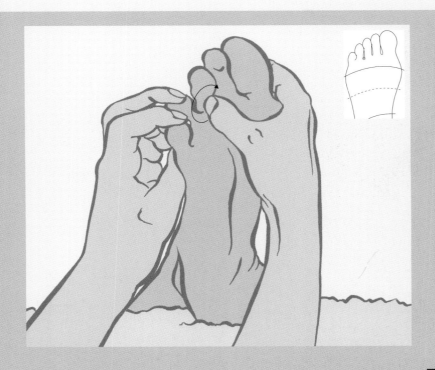

12 To treat the reflex area to the **ears,** thumb-walk from the eustachian tube reflex across the base of the fourth and fifth toe.

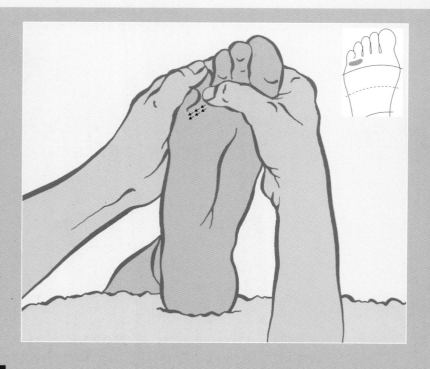

13 The **thyroid gland** reflex is found over the top half of the ball of the big toe. Supporting the top of the foot with your left hand, thumb-walk over this area with your working hand, using semi-circular movements.

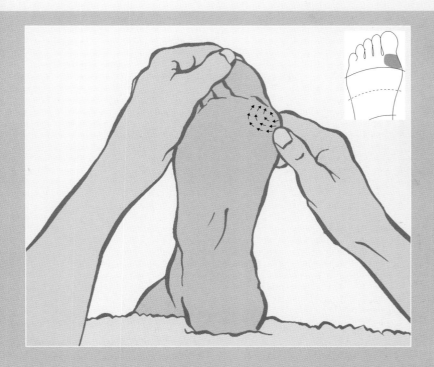

14 Without changing the position of your hands, work the first
parathyroid area, at the base of the big toe. Place your working
thumb on the lateral edge of the thyroid reflex and gently rotate
for a few seconds.

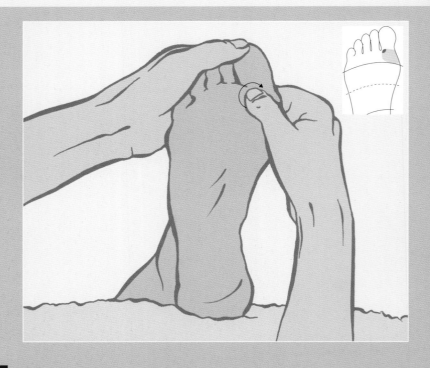

15 Still supporting the top of the foot, move your working thumb to the base of the lateral aspect of the thyroid gland and continue the rotary movement on the second **parathyroid** area.

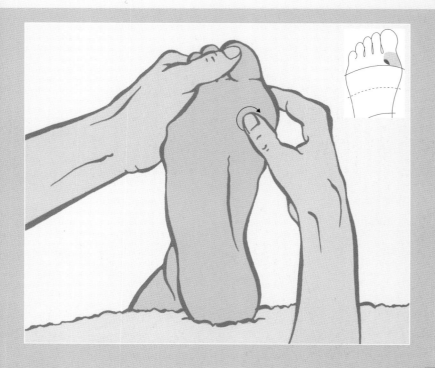

16 Now work the **teeth** reflexes on the fronts of the second, third, fourth and fifth toes. Change the position of your hands by moving the supporting left hand down to the middle part of the foot. Finger-walk with the working right hand across the fronts of the second and third toes. Change hands once more to finger-walk across the fourth and fifth toes.

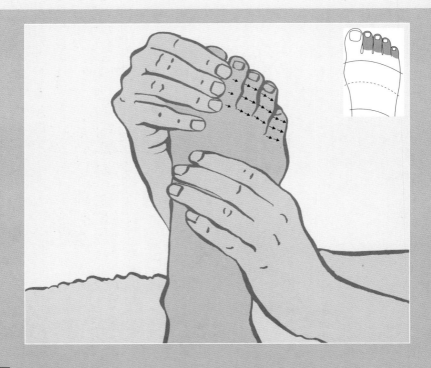

Shoulder and chest reflexes

The shoulder and chest reflexes are located on both feet. They are situated between the first transverse zone line and the diaphragm, an area which ranges from the base of the toes to the diaphragm. (The best way to locate the diaphragm is to visualize a line starting at the lower end of the ball of the big toe and extending across the sole of the foot.)

Start with the shoulder reflex, followed by the reflexes to the arm and elbow, the trachea, the bronchi into the lungs, the thymus gland, the heart, sternum and ribs, and complete this section with the diaphragm. Remember that the heart reflex is found on the left foot only, and will therefore be worked when treating the left side of the body. Take note of any reflexes that feel abnormal, so that you can return to them and give them additional treatment after both feet have been worked. When you treat the lung area, you may find that it feels gritty: this could be down to the level of pollution in the air, or excessive smoking. With regular treatment, this can be cleared. When you find a reflex to be painful, only apply light, continuous pressure so as not to cause undue discomfort.

SHOULDER
The shoulder is a ball-and-socket joint held in place largely by the muscles that move it. The joint is formed by the bone of the upper arm, or humerus, and the shoulder blade, or scapula. Pain in the shoulder can be caused by many conditions not originating in the joint itself. Some of the causes of pain are arthritis of the joint, tendinitis, bursitis, supraspinatus syndrome and frozen shoulder.

ARM AND ELBOW
The arm is made up of the humerus bone, which links the shoulder joint to the elbow joint; the radius and ulna bones, linking the elbow to the

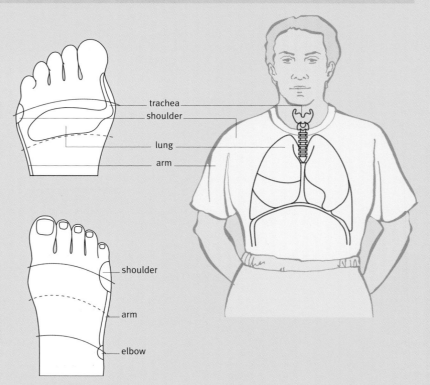

trachea
shoulder
lung
arm

shoulder

arm

elbow

Reflexes on the right foot correspond to organs and muscles on the right side of the body, and those on the left foot, to the left side. For example, the lung reflex shown here relates to the right lung, the arm reflex to the right arm, and so on.

wrist; and the hand, which is joined to the forearm by the wrist. Problems helped through this reflex include tennis elbow, arthritis and any aches or pains related to this part of the body.

TRACHEA

The trachea, or windpipe, is an air tube about 12 centimetres (5 inches) long and 2.5 centimetres (1 inch) in diameter. It lies in front of the oesophagus and ends opposite the fourth thoracic vertebra – approximately level with the top of the heart. Here it divides into two bronchi, one going to the right lung and the other to the left lung.

The trachea consists of a number of C-shaped rings of cartilage which prevent its walls from collapsing and so keep the windpipe permanently open. The upper four rings of the trachea are crossed by the isthmus of the thyroid gland. The isthmus is a thin strand of thyroid tissue which joins the two lobes of the thyroid gland. Each of the two bronchi divides and subdivides into smaller bronchial tubes to form what is sometimes called the bronchial tree.

LUNGS

The two lungs lie side by side in the chest cavity. They are cone-shaped and greyish in colour. The left lung is slightly smaller than the right and is divided into two lobes by a deep fissure. The right lung is divided into three lobes. Each lung is encased in a thin membrane, the pleura. The bronchial tube leading into each lung divides into bronchioles, which terminate in tiny air sacs called alveoli, giving the lungs the appearance of a sponge.

When we breathe in, the cavity of the thorax is enlarged, and the lungs, being elastic, expand to fill the increased space. When we breathe out, the thorax returns to its former size and the air is expelled from the lungs. It's important to take in air through the nose because the nose contains tiny fibres that act as air filters. This reflex is important for all conditions related to the lungs.

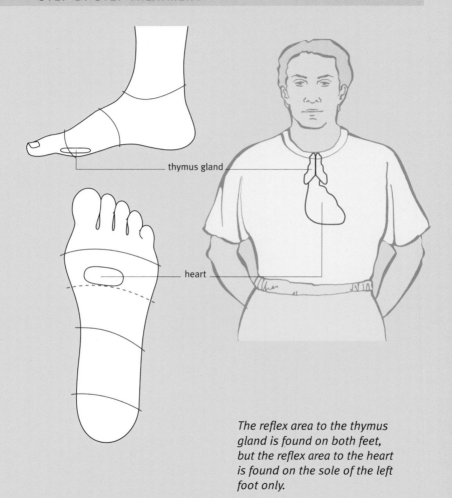

thymus gland

heart

The reflex area to the thymus gland is found on both feet, but the reflex area to the heart is found on the sole of the left foot only.

THYMUS GLAND

The thymus gland is situated in the thoracic cavity, posterior to the sternum and in front of the heart, between the lungs. It consists largely of lymphoid tissue and plays a part in the formation of lymphocytes – a type of white blood cell. At birth this gland is relatively large, and it continues to increase in size until puberty, helping to develop the immune system. After puberty it gradually becomes smaller. The lymphocytes produced in infancy are coded to recognize and protect the body's tissues.

The thymus reflex is important when the immune system is not functioning correctly, especially in children who have not yet reached puberty.

HEART

The heart is a cone-shaped organ made almost entirely of muscle, and is the centre of the circulatory system. It lies roughly in the centre of the chest, two-thirds of it to the left of the breastbone and the other third to the right. Basically, the heart consists of two pumps side by side. Blood is pumped from the right side of the heart to the lungs, where waste gases are removed and oxygen added. Freshly oxygenated blood returns to the left side of the heart, from which it is pumped to all organs and tissues. This requires considerable effort, which is why the left side of the heart is bigger and more powerful than the right. The heart reflex is important for all heart and circulatory problems.

RIBS

Twelve pairs of ribs make up the sides of the thoracic cavity. The upper seven pairs are joined to the sternum by a strip of cartilage and are known as true ribs. The next three pairs do not join the sternum directly and are called false ribs. The eleventh and twelfth pairs are not attached to the sternum and are known as floating ribs. All the ribs are attached to and articulate with the spine.

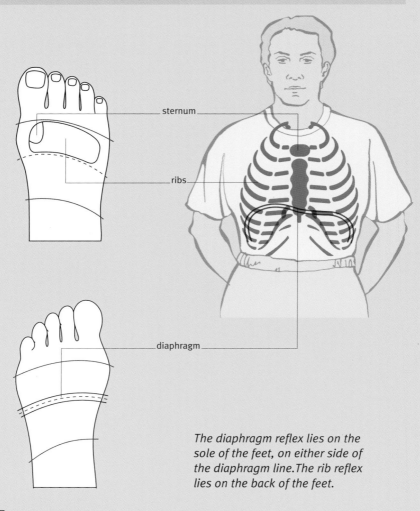

sternum

ribs

diaphragm

The diaphragm reflex lies on the sole of the feet, on either side of the diaphragm line. The rib reflex lies on the back of the feet.

STERNUM

The sternum, or breastbone, is a flat, narrow bone measuring about 15 centimetres (6 inches) in length. It is situated in the median line of the anterior thoracic wall, and attached to it are the ribs and the muscles. The reflexes to both the ribs and the sternum are important where damage has occured in these areas.

DIAPHRAGM

The diaphragm is a large, dome-shaped partition separating the cavity of the thorax from that of the abdomen, and is involved in respiration. It consists partly of muscle and partly of membrane and is attached to the circumference of the thoracic cavity: in front of the lower end of the sternum; on either side, to the lower six ribs; and at the back, to the first two lumbar vertebrae. It is drawn downwards until it's flat during inhalation. During exhalation, the diaphragm and chest muscles relax. This reflex is important in cases of hiatus hernia, and for respiratory problems.

1   Start this part of your treatment with the **shoulder** reflex. This is located in the base and lateral side of the little toe. Supporting the foot with your right hand, place the thumb of your working hand at the lateral edge of the base of the little toe. Thumb-walk several times in semi-circles over this reflex, making sure that you cover the whole area. If your patient is experiencing shoulder pain, work a little longer over the reflex.

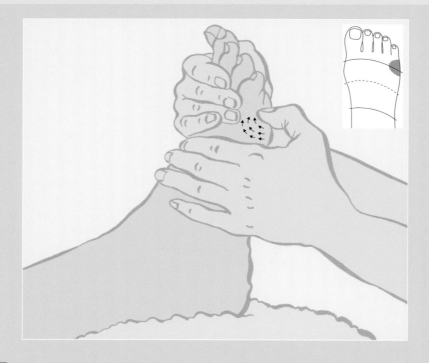

2   The **arm and elbow** reflex extends from the shoulder reflex along the
    lateral edge of the fifth metatarsal bone on the side and top of the
    foot. Change over hands, so that your supporting hand rests just above
    the ankle joint. Place the fingers of your right hand over the top of the
    foot. Starting at the lateral edge, thumb-walk down the reflex; then
    change hands to thumb-walk back up the reflex with your left hand.

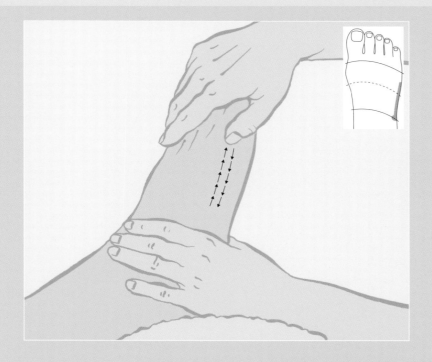

3 Supporting the foot and toes with your left hand, work the **trachea** reflex. Thumb-walk from the medial side of the big toe base, along the medial edge of the ball.

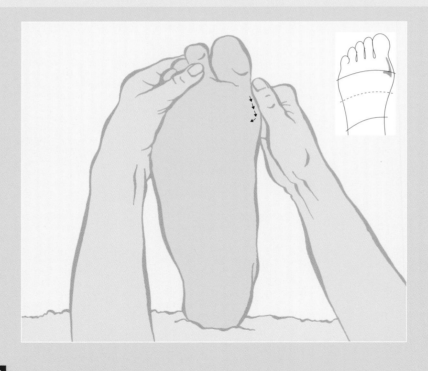

4 The reflex area for the **right lung** is found in all five zones of the right foot. The left lung reflex is on the left foot. Thumb-walk in horizontal lines across this reflex.

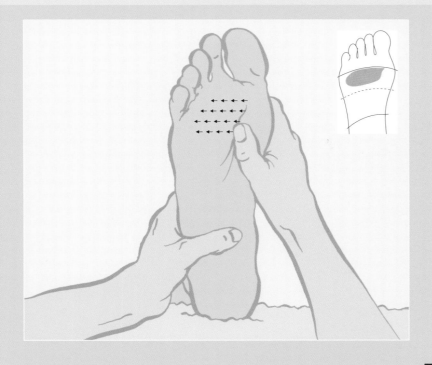

5　To treat the **thymus gland,** change hands and wrap your supporting hand around the heel of the foot, with the thumb on the medial side. With your left hand, gently flex the foot towards you. Place the outer edge of your left thumb onto the front of the foot in zone one. Starting from the medial side at the base of the big toe, thumb-walk down the front of the foot to the end of the third phalanges. This reflex is part of the immune system, playing its biggest role before puberty.

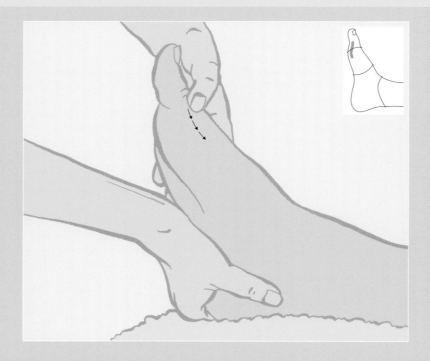

6   The **heart** reflex area is found on the left foot only. Support the foot
    with your right hand. Thumb-walk from the metatarsal bone, covering
    zones two and three.

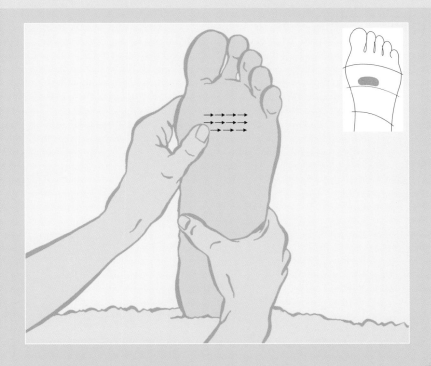

7   Move your working fingers to the **rib** reflex on the top of the foot,
    your thumb supporting on the sole. From the fifth metatarsal bone,
    finger-walk across the foot.

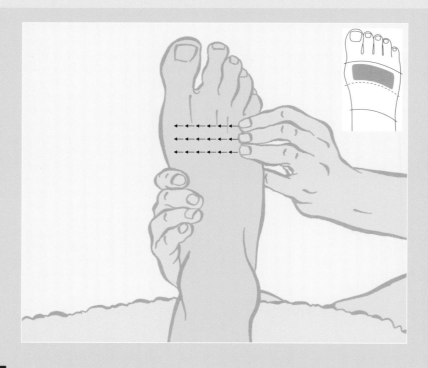

8   Support the foot with your left hand, and place your right thumb
    below the base of the big toe on the top of the foot, in zone one.
    Gently thumb-walk around this area to treat the **sternum** reflex.

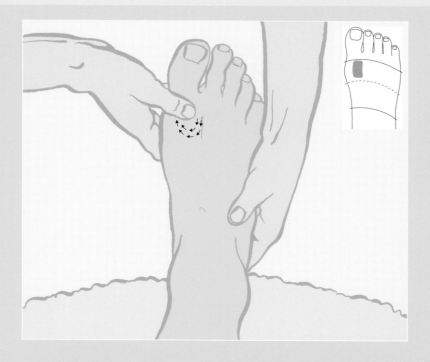

9   To complete this section of the foot, use your right thumb to walk across the **diaphragm** reflex. This area lies either side of a line drawn across the foot, starting beneath the ball of the big toe.

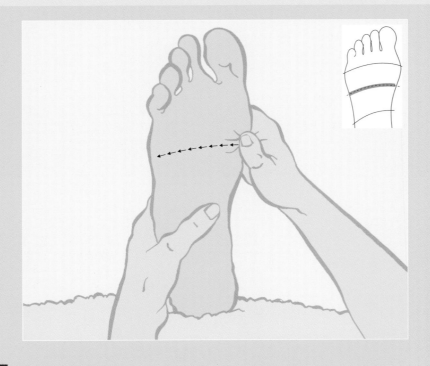

Abdomen reflexes

The reflexes to the abdomen are found beneath the diaphragm in the second and third transverse zones, either side of the waist line on the sole of the foot. These zones cover the lower half of the metatarsals to the upper part of the calcaneum. They include all the organs which constitute the digestive system, and their functions are described below.

Other organs found in the abdomen have been included under lower body reflexes (*see page 96*), since they are located mainly on the medial and lateral borders of the feet. These reflexes would therefore be treated only after completing treatment on the soles of the feet.

SOLAR PLEXUS
The anterior branches of the spinal nerves (except for two of them) don't go directly to the structures of the body they supply. Instead, they form networks on either side of the body by joining with adjacent nerves. Such a network is called a plexus. The solar plexus – resembling sun rays – is situated behind the stomach. It is an important reflex wherever stress or tension is present.

LIVER
The liver is the largest solid organ of the body. It is situated in the upper part of the abdomen, beneath the diaphragm and mainly on the right side of the body. It is divided into a large right lobe and a smaller tapering left lobe. The liver undertakes many chemical activities. It neutralizes toxic substances from the small intestine, produces bile which assists digestion, and stores vitamins and glycogen; it manufactures enzymes, cholesterol, complex proteins, vitamin A and blood coagulation factors; and it is also involved in carbohydrate, fat and protein metabolism. This is an important reflex where the body is overly toxic, and for diseases such as hepatitis and jaundice.

GALL BLADDER

The gall bladder is a sac of approximately 7.5 centimetres (3 inches) in length, found on the undersurface of the right lobe of the liver. Its function is to store and concentrate the bile, secreted by the liver, that helps break down fatty foods. In order to participate in the digestive process, bile is ejected, by muscle contraction, through the bile duct and into the small intestine. This is an important reflex for gallstones and in conditions where the digestion of fat is difficult.

SPLEEN

The spleen is a very large lymph gland lying on the upper left side of the abdomen. In addition to producing lymphocytes – a type of white blood cell – the spleen also removes old and malformed red cells from the bloodstream and breaks them down. This is an important reflex when building up defence against infection.

OESOPHAGUS

The oesophagus is a muscular tube that runs from the back of the throat, through the neck and chest, to the stomach. After swallowing, food passes along this tube to the stomach by rhythmic contractions of the oesophageal muscles. Situated at the base of the oesophagus is a muscular valve which relaxes and opens to allow food into the stomach, but also prevents the acid contents of the stomach from flowing back into the oesophagus, where they can cause irritation. This is an important reflex where there is difficulty in swallowing.

STOMACH

The stomach is located behind the lower ribs, mainly to the left side of the body. When food enters the stomach from the oesophagus, powerful muscles in the stomach wall start to crush and mix it with the hydrochloric acid and digestive enzymes manufactured there. The main digestive enzyme is pepsin, which breaks down protein foods such as meat. This enzyme is only active when there is acid present. The semi-digested food

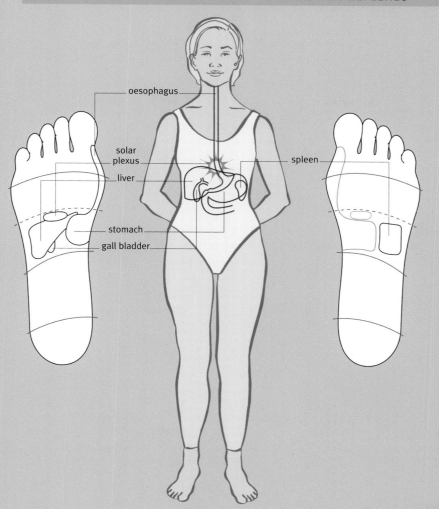

oesophagus

solar plexus

liver

spleen

stomach

gall bladder

then passes through the pyloric sphincter into the duodenum. The stomach reflex is important for problems relating to the stomach, such as ulcers, cancer, indigestion and heartburn, and for general digestive problems.

PANCREAS

The pancreas lies behind the stomach. Part of the endocrine system, it is a double-purpose gland with many branched ducts. Its small clusters of islet cells secrete insulin, a hormone that is essential for utilizing sugars, and without which diabetes may develop. Many of the foods we eat contain glucose, the main source of energy for all the cells in our body. Insulin stimulates those cells to absorb enough glucose from the blood for the energy they need. It then activates the liver to absorb and store the surplus. The mass of pancreatic cells produces pancreatic juices, which pass along the pancreatic duct into the duodenum, where they help break down carbohydrates, proteins and fats. The pancreas reflex is important for certain digestive disorders, for hyper- and hypoglycaemia, and for diabetes.

SMALL INTESTINE

The small intestine is a tube about 5 to 6 metres (17 to 20 feet) long and is divided into the duodenum, the jejunum and the ileum. It is the main site for the absorption of nutrients into the bloodstream. The semi-digested food from the stomach passes into the duodenum, where the digestive process is furthered by the secretion of enzymes, bile from the gall bladder and pancreatic juice from the pancreas. Food is pushed along the small intestine by peristaltic waves of contractions of the muscles in its walls. Once the food molecules are small enough, they pass through the thin lining of the intestine into the bloodstream and then on to the liver for storage and distribution. The small intestine reflex is important for all diseases affecting the digestive tract. Disorders of this type include Crohn's disease, coeliac disease and digestive problems.

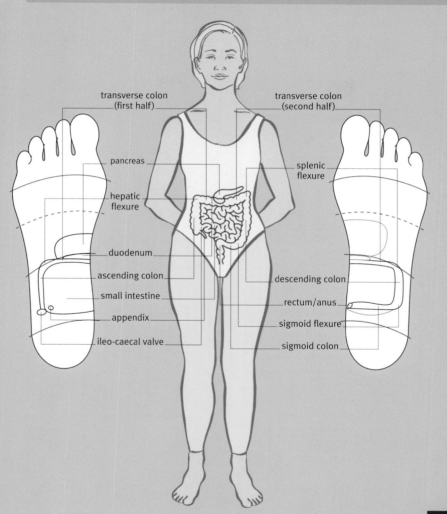

transverse colon
(first half)

transverse colon
(second half)

pancreas

splenic
flexure

hepatic
flexure

duodenum

ascending colon

descending colon

small intestine

rectum/anus

appendix

sigmoid flexure

ileo-caecal valve

sigmoid colon

APPENDIX

The appendix is a thin worm-shaped pouch, about 7.5 centimetres (3 inches) long, that projects from the first part of the large intestine. In herbivorous animals the appendix is relatively large compared with its size in humans, and it plays an important role in the digestive process. In the human body, the appendix is considered to be an evolutionary relic. It is an important reflex where there is suspected appendicitis.

ILEO-CAECAL VALVE

The ileo-caecal valve is a fold of mucous membrane which guards the opening from the ileum to the large intestine. It allows materials from the small intestine to pass into the large intestine and prevents a backflow from the large to small intestine. This is an important reflex in cases of constipation.

LARGE INTESTINE (COLON)

The large intestine is about 1.5 metres (5 feet) long and consists of two main organs: the colon and the rectum. The colon is divided into several sections. The ascending colon ascends on the right side of the abdomen to the undersurface of the liver. Here it bends to the left (hepatic flexure) and continues as the transverse colon, across the abdomen to the lower end of the spleen. At this point it curves (splenic flexure) and passes down the left side of the body as the descending colon. The last section is the sigmoid colon. It projects inwards to the midline and terminates as the rectum. The rectum is a short tube of about 12.5 centimetres (5 inches) in length leading to the anus.

Fluid and various mineral salts from the intestinal contents are absorbed into the bloodstream through the membranous wall of the colon. The semi-solid faeces that remain move down into the rectum, from where they are eventually excreted as stools. This reflex is important in cases of constipation, irritable bowel syndrome, diverticulosis, ulcerative colitis and diarrhoea.

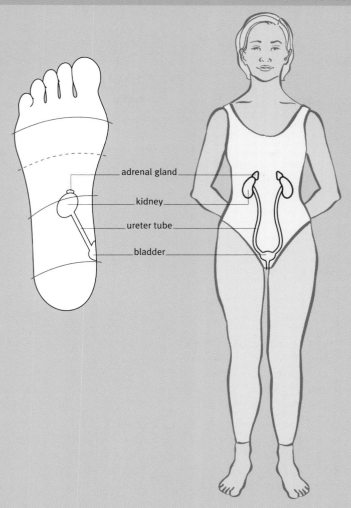

adrenal gland

kidney

ureter tube

bladder

BLADDER

The urinary bladder is a hollow muscular organ situated in the pelvic cavity. Its function is to store urine, which trickles down the ureter tubes from the kidneys. In a male the bladder is directly anterior to the rectum; in a female it is anterior to the vagina and inferior to the uterus. The bladder has elastic flexible walls which allow it to expand as it fills and then contract through the relaxed sphincter muscle when urinating. When the bladder contracts, urine is prevented from flowing back up the ureter tubes by valves that link the ureter tubes to the bladder. The urine is expelled from the bladder through the urethra. The male urethra, which is longer than the female one, also provides an outlet for semen. The bladder reflex is important for all conditions related to the urinary tract – for example, cystitis.

URETER TUBES

The body has two ureter tubes, each approximately 25 to 30 centimetres (10 to 12 inches) long. The purpose of these tubes is to carry urine from the kidneys to the bladder. The reflexes to the ureter tubes are important when kidney stones are present, and for all infections to the urinary system.

KIDNEYS

The kidneys are bean-shaped, deep maroon in colour and weigh about 150 grams (5 ounces) They are approximately 10 centimetres (4 inches) long and 5 centimetres (2 inches) wide, and are situated above the waist on either side of the spinal column, below the lowest ribs. The right kidney, which lies just below the liver, is usually lower than the left. Both kidneys are surrounded by fat, which cushions and supports them.

The kidneys receive their blood supply from the renal artery. This artery divides into progressively smaller branches which infiltrate the kidney tissue and filtering units. The blood is collected by an intricate system of small veins, which join to form larger vessels that empty into the renal vein, returning blood to the general circulation. Kidney cells also manufacture substances that help to control blood pressure. When the blood supply to the kidneys is diminished, these substances are manufactured in larger amounts, and cause raised blood pressure in an attempt to increase the blood flow through the kidneys. Each kidney contains over one million tiny filtering units, called glomeruli, which remove waste chemicals and excess water from the blood travelling through them. The filtered liquid passes from the glomeruli to the central section of the kidney along a long thin tubule, which is surrounded by blood vessels. These blood vessels reabsorb the nutrients from the liquid. The remaining urine continues along the tubule into the ureter and into the bladder. This is a very important reflex for infections and for all problems relating to the urinary system.

ADRENAL GLANDS

The adrenal glands are two small triangular bodies lying just above the kidneys. They consist of the medulla, which forms the inner portion of the gland, and the cortex, which forms the outer part composed of layered glandular cells. The medulla secretes adrenaline and noradrenaline, which is vital in energizing the body to meet sudden dangers and alarms and also plays an important part in controlling heart rate and blood pressure. The cortex secretes steroid hormones, which are closely linked in structure but differing in activity. The adrenal reflexes are important in cases of hormonal imbalance, stress, arthritis, asthma and allergies.

1 Holding and supporting the toes with your left hand, press the **solar plexus** reflex with the thumb of your working hand. This reflex lies just below the diaphragm line, between the second and third zones. Gently rotate on this point in a clockwise direction.

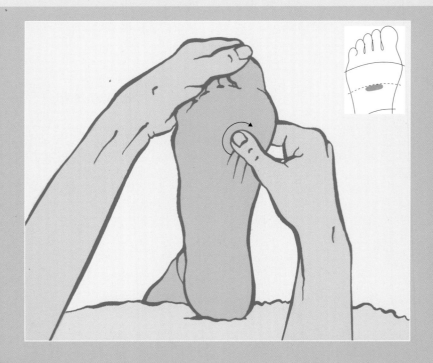

2   The **liver** reflex is found only on the right foot and looks similar to an unequal-sided triangle. Its longest side sits just below the diaphragm and covers all five zones. Its shortest side lies between the diaphragm and the waist line. Holding the foot with your right hand, bend the toes back slightly to open up the reflex areas. With the outer edge of your left thumb, walk horizontally across the reflex, following the shape of the triangle.

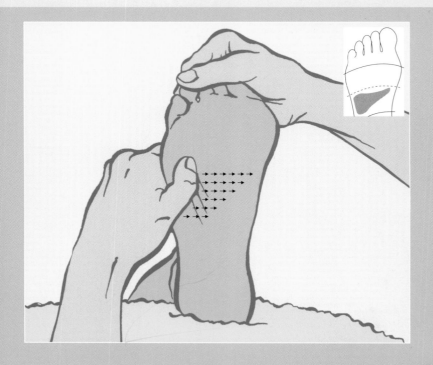

3 Without moving your supporting hand, locate the **gall bladder** reflex. This is found on the right foot only and lies in zone three, just below the liver reflex, and approximately one finger's width above the waist line. Although this is an important reflex, it's also very small and sometimes difficult to find, so you may find it helpful to consult the chart of reflexes. Then, with your working thumb, rotate in an anticlockwise direction.

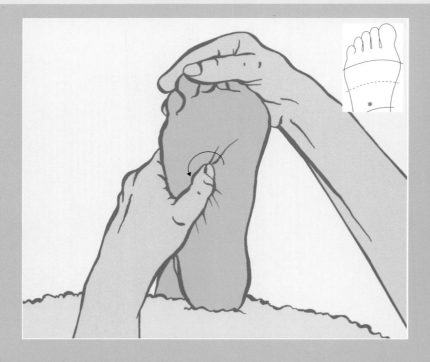

4   The **splenic** reflex is found only on the left foot. It lies in zones four
    and five, below the diaphragm and just above the waist line. Change
    the position of your hands so that your right hand becomes the
    working one. Holding the foot with your left hand, bend the toes back
    slightly. Thumb-walk with your working hand across this area in
    horizontal lines.

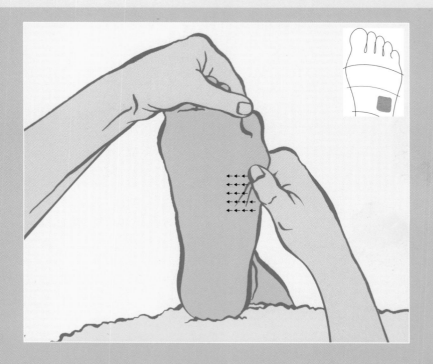

5 The reflex for the **oesophagus** is worked prior to treating the stomach reflex. This is found on the medial side of the foot in zone one, leading down from the big toe to just below the diaphragm. Supporting the heel of the foot with your right hand, thumb-walk down this reflex.

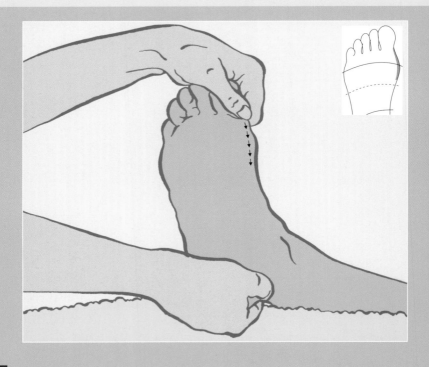

6   From the oesophagus, continue the treatment by working on the reflex
    to the **stomach**. This is found on both feet, between the diaphragm
    and the waist line. On the right foot, the reflex area covers zone one.
    On the left foot it covers zones one, two and three. Bending back the
    toes with your supporting hand, thumb-walk horizontally across this
    area with your working hand.

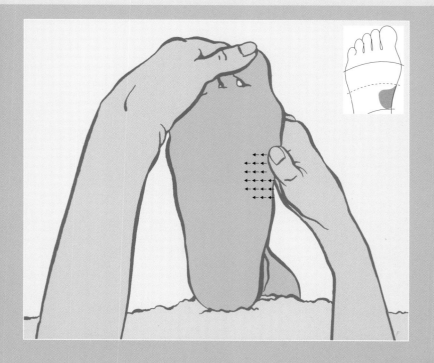

7   Still supporting the foot with your left hand, move your working
    hand one thumb's width below the ball of the big toe so that you can
    thumb-walk across the **pancreas** reflex. This extends to the waist line
    and covers zones one, two and three on the left foot and zones one
    and two on the right foot.

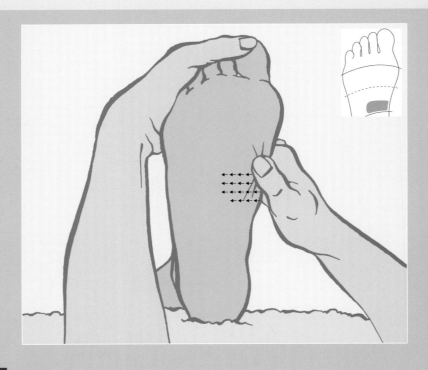

8   With your supporting hand, bend the toes back to help you locate the tendon on the sole of the foot. Then move your working thumb down in zone one to the medial side of this tendon, where it crosses the waist line. This is the **duodenum** reflex. Rotate gently on this point in a clockwise direction.

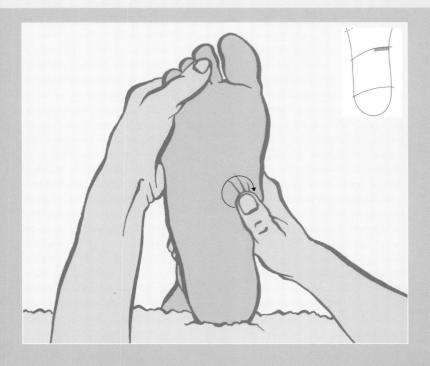

9 The reflex area for the **small intestine** lies on the medial side of the foot below the waist line, at the start of the tarsal bones, and covers zones one to four on both feet. With your right thumb, walk across the top of this reflex. Then change hands and thumb-walk back with your left hand. Cover the whole area.

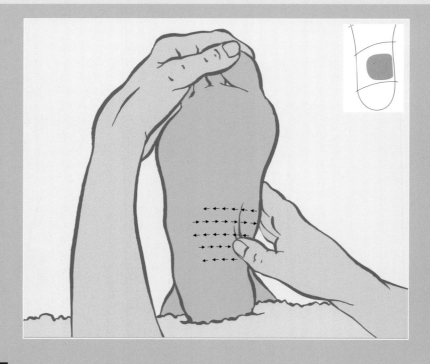

10   Now find the **appendix** reflex. This is located over the tarsal bones in zone four, just above the pelvic girdle, on the right foot only. With the thumb of your right hand, slowly rotate on this reflex in a clockwise direction.

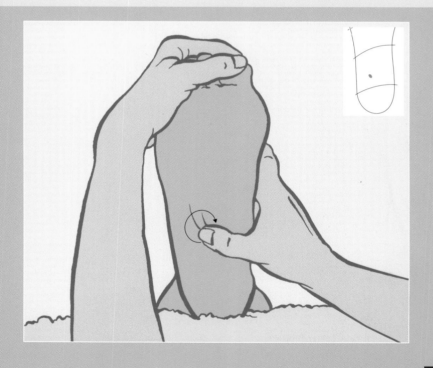

11 Next to the appendix reflex, in zones four and five, you will find the reflex for the **ileo-caecal valve**. Without changing the position of your hands, gently rotate on this point with your working thumb, then continue to thumb-walk up the foot in zones four and five to waist level, to treat the **ascending colon** reflex. When you have reached waist level, press three or four times on that point to treat the **hepatic flexure**. (NOTE: these reflexes are found on the right foot only.)

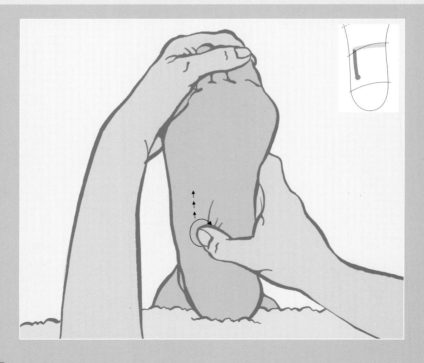

12 To treat the **transverse colon,** start with the first half, which lies
    on the right side of the body (the first part of the transverse colon
    reflex area is thus found on the right foot). Change hands from the
    previous step, and thumb-walk at waist level across all five zones.

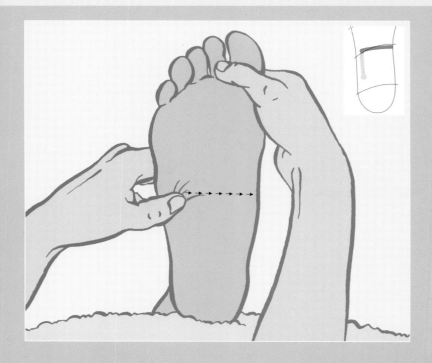

13 The remainder of the **transverse colon** is found on the left foot. Treat it when you work that foot. Thumb-walk across to the medial border of zone five, where the **splenic flexure** is found. Gently press two or three times on this point.

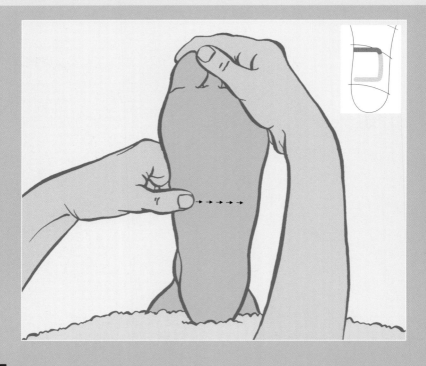

14 To work the reflex area for the **descending colon**, support the foot with your left hand. Thumb-walk in zones four and five to the base of the calcaneum, and press on the **sigmoid flexure** a few times. (NOTE: these reflexes, and those in steps 15 and 16, are found on the left foot only, and should therefore be treated when you treat the left foot.)

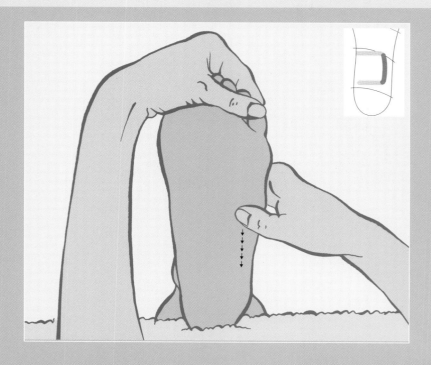

15 Without changing hands, thumb-walk across the foot to the **sigmoid colon** reflex on the medial side of zone one. If your patient suffers from constipation, this reflex may feel lumpy and tender.

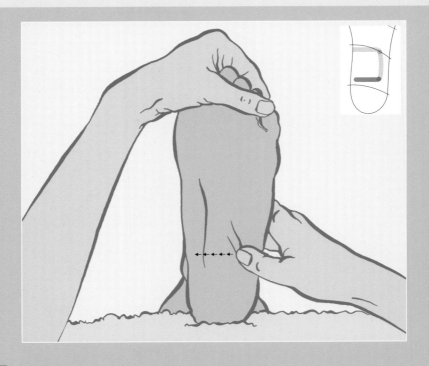

16 When your thumb has reached the medial side of zone one, slowly rotate on this point, in an anticlockwise direction, for a few seconds. This is the reflex for the **rectum and anus**. The rectum is linked to the anus by the anal canal.

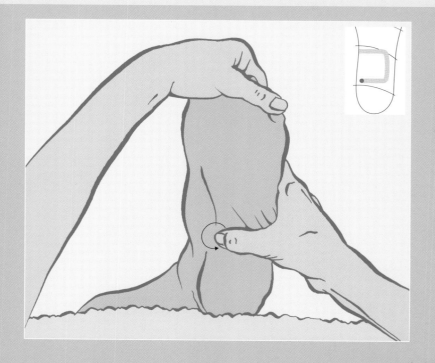

17 Supporting the heel of the foot with your working hand, use your
working thumb to walk over the **bladder** reflex, the slightly puffy
area found on the medial side of the foot.

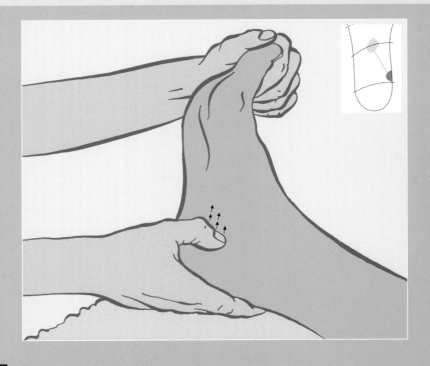

18 From the bladder reflex, thumb-walk up the **ureter tube** reflex, across zones two and three, to waist level. The easiest way to find this reflex is to gently bend the toes back and follow the path of the tendon.

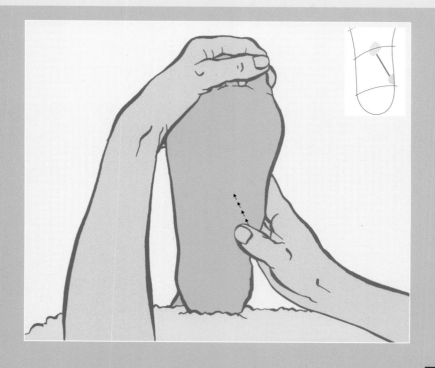

19 You will find the reflex to the **right kidney** at the end of the ureter
    tube, in zones two and three, at waist level. With your working
    thumb, slowly rotate on this point in a clockwise direction.

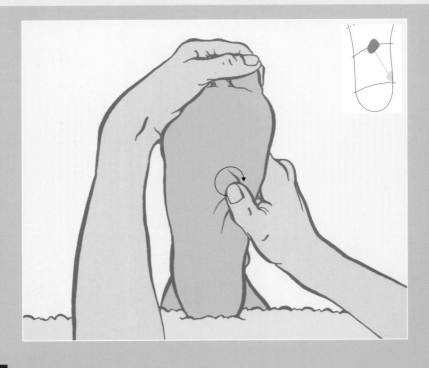

20 Close to the kidney reflex in zone two, just above the waist level, is the reflex to the **right adrenal gland**. Move your working thumb to this position and work this point with a rotating movement.

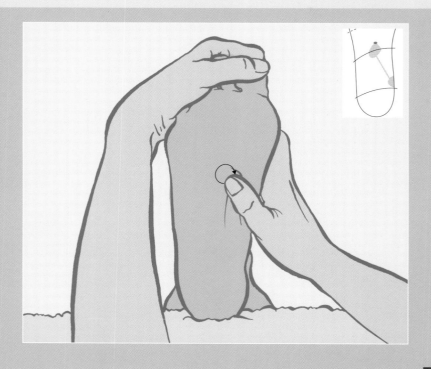

Lower body reflexes

The reflexes to the lower body are often included in the description of abdominal reflexes, since they relate to organs found in the abdomen. However, none of them has any digestive function. Furthermore, with the exception of the sciatic nerve reflex, which crosses the sole of the foot and continues up the back of the leg, on either side of the Achilles tendon, they are all found on the lateral and medial sides of the feet. Therefore treatment of these reflexes comes after treatment of the reflexes located on the soles of the feet.

The lower body reflexes consist of the sciatic nerve, sacro-iliac joint, pelvic muscles, knee, hip, and both the male and female reproductive organs. They are important for chronic ailments associated with these areas. The reproductive reflexes can be tender and therefore should always be treated gently. Great care should also be exercised with the reproductive organs during the first sixteen weeks of pregnancy. These should not be treated if there is a history of miscarriage.

SCIATIC NERVE
The sciatic nerve is the largest nerve in the body and supplies all the muscles of the legs and feet. It arises from the sacral plexus, runs from the spine across the buttocks, and down the back of each leg. Just above the knee, it divides into two branches which supply the lower leg. Pressure exerted on the sciatic nerve – often caused by a 'slipped disc' – produces sciatica, a burning pain radiating through the buttocks and down the back of the thigh. Working with the sciatic reflex can help relieve lower back pain.

SACRO-ILIAC JOINT
This is an important joint transmitting the weight of the body, through the vertebral column, via the pelvis to the lower limbs. It is formed by the

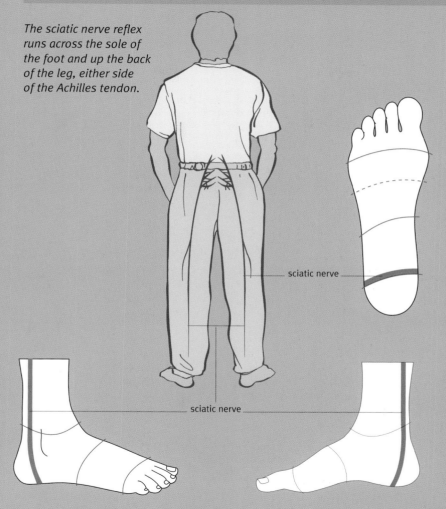

The sciatic nerve reflex runs across the sole of the foot and up the back of the leg, either side of the Achilles tendon.

sciatic nerve

sciatic nerve

sacrum and the ilium and has very little movement. The reflex for this joint is important in cases of sciatica and for lower back or hip problems.

PELVIC MUSCLES

The pelvis is continuous with the abdominal cavity. It is a big funnel-shaped ring of bone formed by the sacrum and coccyx, the pubic bones and the ischium. In all humans, the pelvis joins the legs to the spine in such a way as to maintain the upright position. In a woman, the pelvis also serves to hold and protect the reproductive organs: the two ovaries lie in the cavity of the pelvis. When a baby is born, it has to pass through the hole in the pelvis. In men this is small and flat, but in women it is round and the size of a baby's head. The muscles related to this part of the body form the pelvic floor, and support the bone structure. The most important of these is the levator ani. The pelvic muscles reflex is important for lower back pain and problems related to the hips and pelvis.

HIP

The hip is a major weight-bearing joint and is located where the pelvis meets the femur (thigh bone). It is a ball-and-socket joint, with a strong capsule surrounding it for strength. This reflex is important for back pain and for hip disorders such as arthritis.

KNEE

The knee is the largest joint in the body and is susceptible to most of the common joint disorders. Stability of the joint depends on the strength and tone of the quadriceps muscles on the front of the thigh, which hold the joint in position. The knee reflex is important for various forms of arthritis, including bursitis, rheumatoid arthritis and osteoarthritis of the knee, and any other problems that may be connected to this part of the body.

TESTES AND VAS DEFERENS

The male sex glands, or testes, lie in the scrotal sac, just below the abdomen. This vulnerable position is necessary because the formation

With the exception of the sciatic nerve, all the lower body reflexes are located on the lateral and medial sides of both feet.

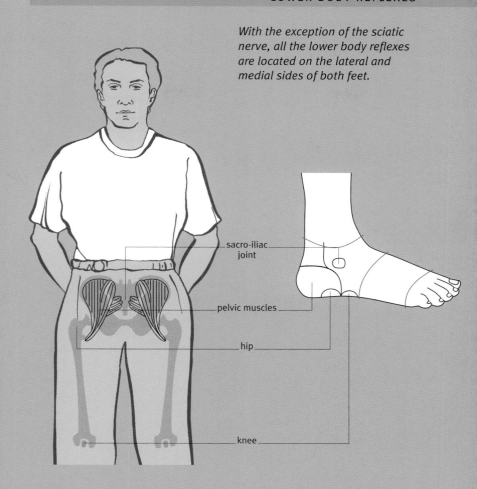

sacro-iliac joint

pelvic muscles

hip

knee

of spermatozoa requires a temperature slightly lower than that found in the abdomen. Each gland is attached to the body by a single spermatic cord composed of the vas deferens, or sperm duct, and a number of nerves and blood vessels. The endocrine part of the testes is composed of clumps of cells that secrete the male hormone, testosterone. They also produce small amounts of the female hormone called oestrogen. The testes are under the control of the hypothalamus and the anterior pituitary gland, and do not develop until puberty.

The sperm produced by each testicle remains in a coiled tube, the epididymis, for approximately three months. After this time the sperm, now mature, passes into the vas deferens and seminal vesicles for storage. There, it swims in the seminal fluid, the volume of which depends on adequate testosterone. If the sperm is not ejaculated with the seminal fluid, it will disintegrate and be reabsorbed into the body.

PROSTATE

The prostate gland comprises three major lobes, which surround the urethra at the point where it leaves the bladder. It is intimately associated with the lower urinary tract. If it becomes enlarged in later life, it can press on the urethra, eventually closing it and making it impossible to pass urine. When this occurs, surgical intervention is necessary. The lobes of the prostate are tubular, with muscles that squeeze their secretions into the urethra, particularly during sexual intercourse. The main disorders that can affect the prostate are enlargement, infections and growths. These can be helped by working the reflex to this gland.

OVARIES, UTERUS AND FALLOPIAN TUBES

The two ovaries and the uterus, which lie in the lower part of the abdomen, are the main female organs of reproduction. The ovaries, part of the endocrine system, are located on either side of the uterus, and are connected to it by a small tube called the fallopian tube. Like the testes, the ovaries have two functions: to produce ova, or female egg cells, and

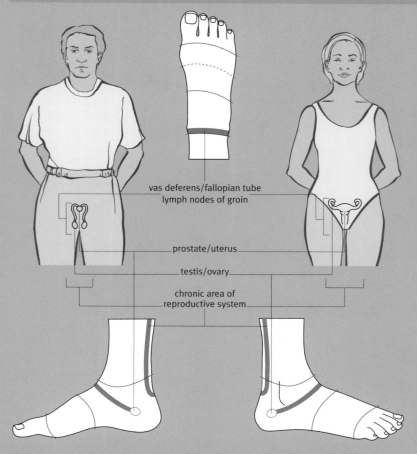

vas deferens/fallopian tube
lymph nodes of groin

prostate/uterus

testis/ovary

chronic area of
reproductive system

The reflexes to the male and female reproductive organs are found across the top of the foot. The uterus or prostate reflex is located on the medial side of the foot, while the ovaries or testes reflex is located on the lateral side.

to produce hormones that change a girl's body into a woman's, and which prepare the uterus for pregnancy. The ovaries waken to activity at puberty through stimulation by the gonadotropins – the hormones secreted by the pituitary gland. In turn, the developing ovarian follicle secretes oestrogen responsible for enlarging the breasts, and for the development of the uterus, the vagina and the rest of the genital tract, at puberty. Halfway through the menstrual cycle, another hormone, prompted by the rising levels of oestrogen, is secreted by the pituitary gland. Under its influence, the developing ovum is released from the ovary, causing the vacated follicle to secrete progesterone. This hormone changes the lining of the uterus in preparation for the eventual reception of a fertilized egg.

The uterus, into which the fertilized ovum becomes embedded, is a hollow, pear-shaped organ about 10 centimetres (4 inches) long, lying between the urinary bladder and the rectum. At the lower end of the uterus is the cervix, the narrow, thick-walled neck which leads into the top of the vagina. After a forty-week gestation period, the fully developed baby enters the world by passing through the dilated cervix and out through the vagina. If pregnancy does not occur, the lining of the uterus breaks down and is discarded through the menstrual flow.

The reflex areas to the reproductive organs in both the male and female are important in cases of infertility, and for all problems associated with those parts of the body.

1 To treat the **sciatic** reflex, wrap the fingers of your right hand around the foot. For added support, hold the front of the foot with your working-hand fingers. Start about one-third down the lateral edge of the heel pad and thumb-walk two parallel lines across it.

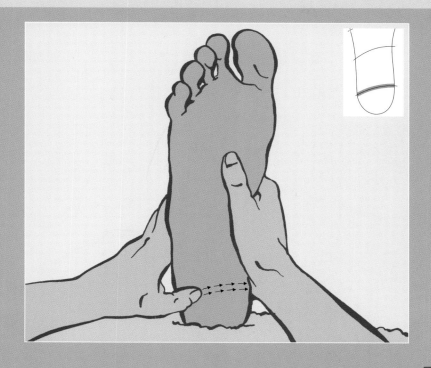

2   Holding the side of the foot and tilting it slightly with your left hand, place your right thumb on the **medial aspect** of the **sciatic** reflex and thumb-walk back up the medial side of the Achilles tendon. Your working-hand fingers will support first the heel, then the leg.

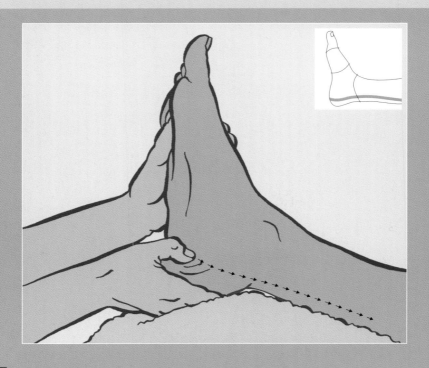

3 Reverse hands and wrap your right hand around the foot (*left*). From the outer edge of the **sciatic** reflex, thumb-walk up the **lateral side** of the Achilles tendon. When you reach the top of the tendon (*right*), place your fingers on the medial side of the sciatic reflex and work back down to the heel, gently squeezing the back of the leg.

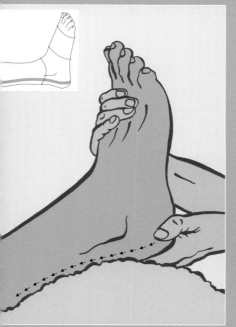

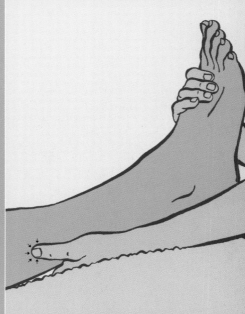

4   Maintaining the supporting position of your right hand, use the thumb of your working hand to gently rotate around the reflex area to the **sacro-iliac joint**. You will find this in the dip which lies just in front of the ankle bone, in line with the fourth toe.

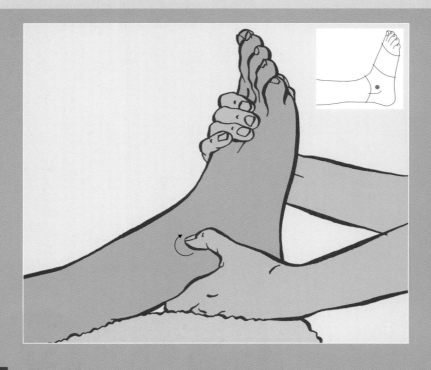

5 The reflex area to the **pelvic muscles** lies on the lateral side of the foot, below the ankle bone. Keep hold of the top of the foot with your right hand and hold the heel with your left. Starting at the base of the ankle bone, walk your left thumb in vertical lines over the reflex area.

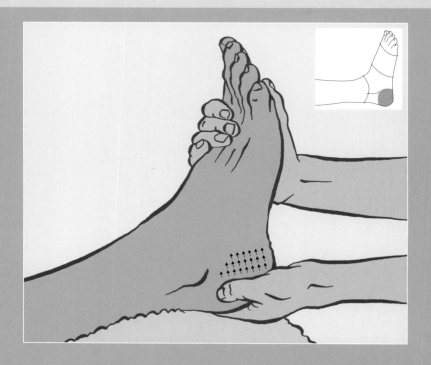

6   Without changing the position of your hands, proceed to the reflex
    areas for the hip and knee. These resemble two half moons and lie on
    the lateral side of the foot, from the end of the metatarsal to a third
    of the way along the calcaneum. The half moon near the calcaneum is
    the **hip** reflex. With the outer edge of your left thumb placed on the
    calcaneum, thumb-walk over this reflex.

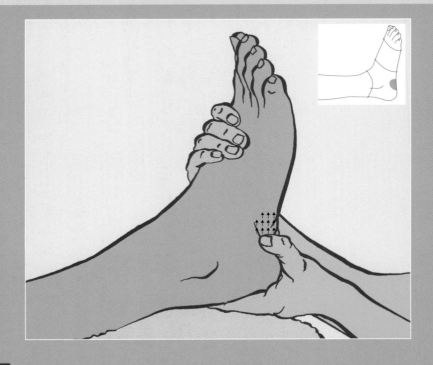

7   The half moon next to the hip reflex is the reflex area to the **knee**.
     Continue your thumb-walking until you have covered the whole
     reflex area.

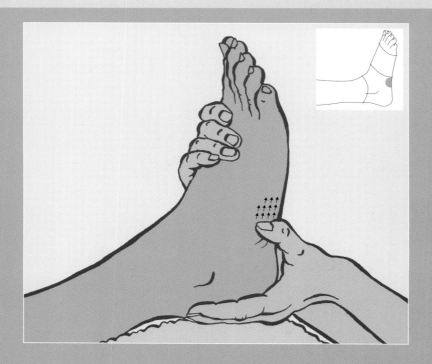

8 Maintaining the same hand positions, tilt your patient's foot slightly to the right with your right hand. The reflex for the **right ovary** or **right testis** lies midway between the outer ankle bone and the back of the heel. Rotate gently with your thumb.

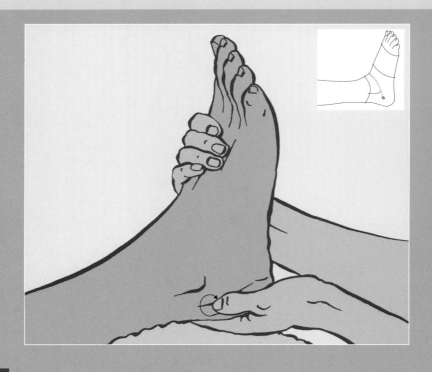

9   From here, thumb-walk across the top of the foot to midway between
    the ankle bone and the back of the heel, on the inner side of the foot.
    This is the area that covers the reflex to the **right fallopian tube** or the
    right vas deferens. The corresponding left reflexes are found on the
    left foot.

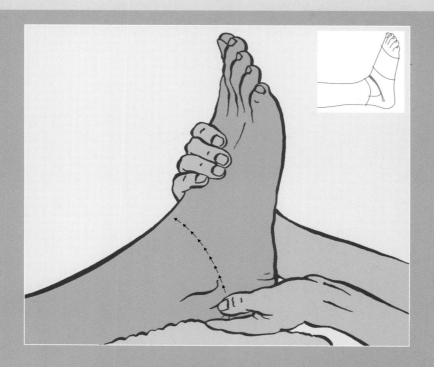

10 To treat the **uterus** or **prostate** reflex, you need to change the positions of your working and supporting hands. Putting your right thumb over the reflex, slowly rotate your thumb around the area. This can be tender, so care is needed.

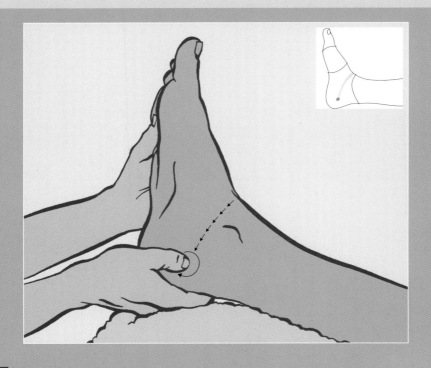

Reflexes on the top of the foot

To complete a reflexology treatment, the remaining reflexes found on the top of the foot are worked. These reflexes are positioned between the base of the toes and the top of the ankle, and comprise the breasts, mid-back and lymphatic system including lymph drainage. When you work on the breast reflexes, feel for any abnormalities, since lumps or cysts in the breasts can be detected in the course of treatment. (Be sure to suggest that your patient seek medical advice if you feel you may have located a problem.) When treating the lymph reflexes, puffiness in these areas may indicate swollen lymph nodes, which means that infection is present in the body.

In elderly people, the veins around the sides and over the top of the foot can sometimes be prominent. If you encounter this, take the utmost care and work very gently over these areas to avoid bruising.

BREASTS

The essential function of the breasts is milk secretion and ejection. The milk secretion is due largely to the hormone called prolactin, with contributions from the progesterone and oestrogen hormones.

Each breast consists of approximately fifteen to twenty groups of milk-producing glands embedded in fatty tissue, which gives the breast its characteristic shape. A milk duct runs to the nipple from each group of glands. Around the nipple is a dark area, the areola, which contains small lubricating glands keeping the nipple supple. The breasts may enlarge as a result of the change in hormone levels, prior to menstruation and also during pregnancy. This reflex is important for disorders of the breast, such as benign or malignant lumps and mastitis.

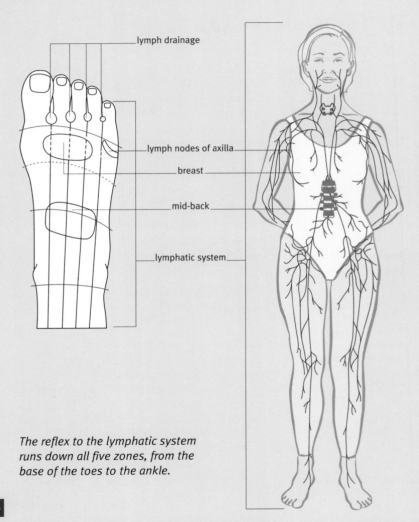

lymph drainage

lymph nodes of axilla

breast

mid-back

lymphatic system

The reflex to the lymphatic system runs down all five zones, from the base of the toes to the ankle.

MID-BACK

The mid-back consists of the area between the tenth thoracic vertebra and the third lumbar vertebra. This reflex is beneficial for all back-related conditions. These include disc problems, muscular aches and strains, and various types of arthritis. When working with any of these disorders, it is advisable to give extra treatment to the spinal reflex as well as the mid-back reflex.

LYMPHATIC SYSTEM

The lymphatic system is widely distributed within the body. It consists of the lymph glands, or nodes, that are found principally in the neck, armpits and groin, and the lymphatics – the small vessels that link them. These contain a watery fluid, called lymph. The lymph nodes secrete very large numbers of lymphocytes, a type of white blood cell, which produce antibodies against recurrent infections. These nodes act as barriers to the spread of infection through the lymphatic vessels.

The lymph carries nutrients and oxygen from the blood to every cell in the body, and drains back into the bloodstream through the lymphatic system. If there is a blockage in the flow of lymph, swelling (oedema) results. The reflex points for all of the lymph nodes are found on the top of the feet. These include the upper lymph nodes and the lymph nodes to the axilla or armpit, the breast, the abdomen, the pelvis and the groin. These reflexes are important in cases of infection. They also help maintain a healthy lymphatic system to protect the body from disease.

LYMPH DRAINAGE

After you have finished treating the lymphatic system, complete this section by working on the lymph drainage reflex. The reflex areas are found on the top of the foot between the toes, the most important area being between the big toe and the second toe.

1   The **breast** reflex is found in all five zones on the top of the foot and
    covers the area between the base of the toes and the diaphragm.
    Support the foot with your right hand. Place your left thumb on the
    sole and, with your fingers on the top of the foot, walk horizontally
    across this reflex with your first three fingers.

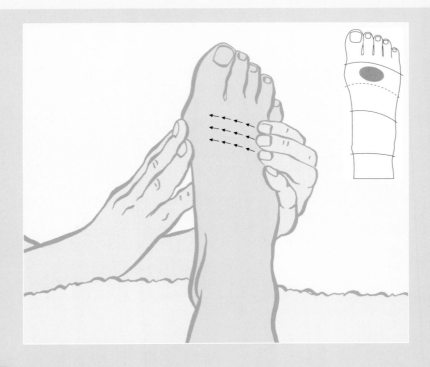

2   Slide your working hand down the foot to the **mid-back** reflex, which is found just below the waist line. Finger-walk horizontally across all five zones to just above the ankle. The thumb of your working hand should remain resting on the sole of the foot, behind your working fingers.

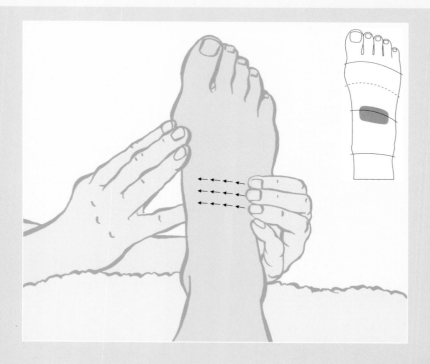

3 Begin treating the lymphatic system with the reflex to the **lymph nodes** of the right armpit, positioned just below the shoulder reflex. With the index finger of your left hand over this reflex, and your thumb on the sole of the foot, slowly rotate for a few seconds.

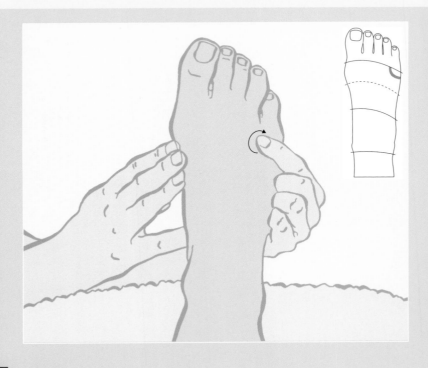

4   The reflex areas to the rest of the **lymphatic system** are on the top of
    the foot, from the webs of the toes to the ankle bone. Support the sole
    of the foot with your left hand. From the web between the first and
    second toe, thumb-walk down zone one. Repeat for all the other zones.

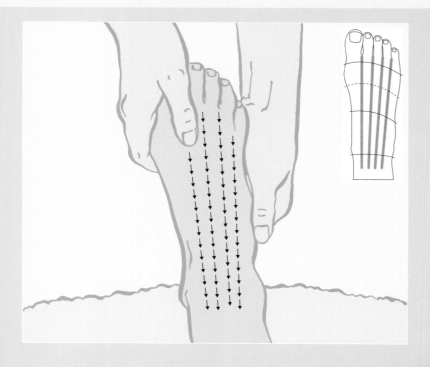

5 The reflex areas for **lymph drainage** are found on the webs between the toes. The most important of these is the web between the first and second toe. Support the foot with your left hand and, with the thumb and index finger of your right hand, pinch and slide off each toe web.

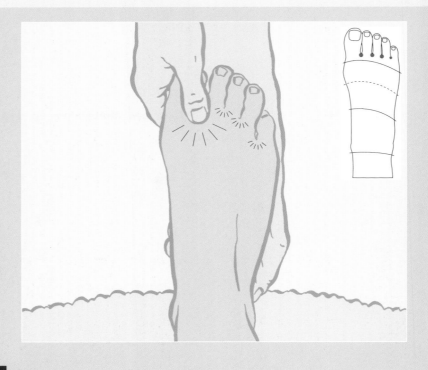

Finishing the treatment

When you have worked all the reflexes on both feet, complete your treatment with foot massage. This relaxes the patient and stimulates energy flow. Massage techniques can also be used on both feet prior to treatment, for people who are tense or under stress. There are five basic strokes: kneading, wringing, stretching, finger-circling and stroking. These techniques are most effective when performed in this order. Follow your own judgement as to how much time you spend on these massage techniques.

1   Position one hand across the top of the foot and place the clenched
    fist of the other on the sole of the foot. Kneading with both hands,
    make circular movements over the entire foot. This is wonderful for
    both stimulating energy and relaxing a person.

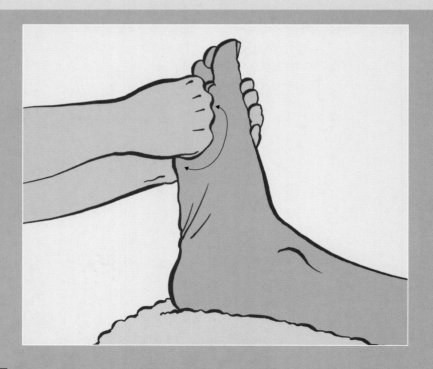

2   Wrap your hands around the sides of the foot near the toes (*left*),
    with your thumbs on the sole. Then, gently twisting your hands back
    and forth in a wringing action (*right*), work your way slowly down
    the foot until you reach the ankle.

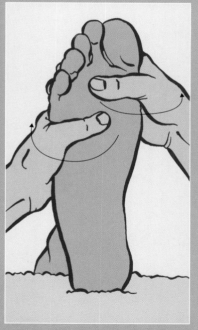
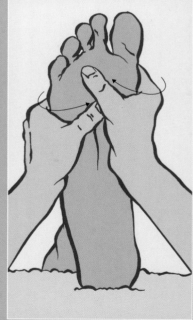

3 Maintain both your hands in the same position. Starting near the ankle, stretch the hands up towards the toes. Repeat several times. This action makes the whole body – especially the spine – feel as though it is being stretched upwards. It is good for people who work sitting at a desk all day.

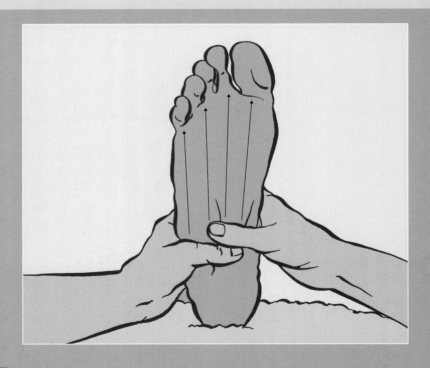

4   Place the fingers of both hands near the toes, and your thumbs on the sole of the foot. Work over the top and sides of the foot and around the ankle bones, using tiny circular movements. This will stimulate the lymphatic system and is the most relaxing of the techniques.

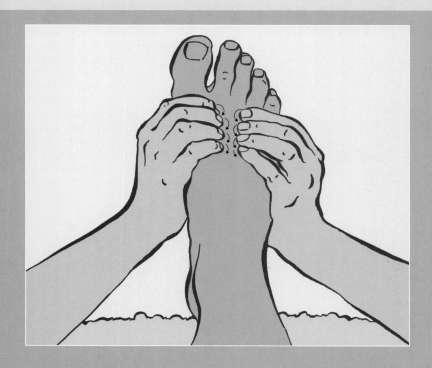

5 Complete your massage by stroking the foot. This stimulates the nerve endings and is a very soothing movement. Starting at the ankle, stroke the top and sides of the feet in a gentle upward movement with the fingers of both hands. Continue for as long as you think necessary.

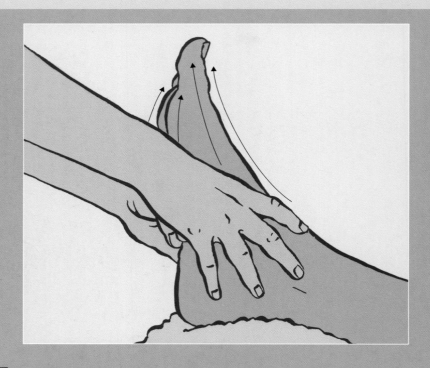

6   When you have massaged both feet, press the palms of your hands against the soles. Visualize a shaft of energizing golden light coming through the top of your head into your hands and being transferred to your patient through their feet.

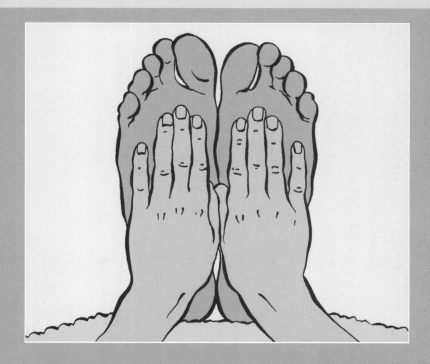

ABOUT THE AUTHOR

Pauline Wills MBRA, H.Dip.C.Th, MIACT, DSA is a qualified reflexologist, colour practitioner and yoga instructor. She has been practising reflexology for over twenty-five years, and pioneered the integration of colour therapy with reflexology. She is co-founder of the Oracle School of Colour in London, where she teaches and practises colour therapy and reflexology, and is the author of a number of books including *Colour Reflexology*, *Colour Therapy* and *Chakra Workbook*. Visit the Oracle School of Colour website at oracleschoolofcolour.com.

EDDISON • SADD EDITIONS

Editorial Director *Ian Jackson*
Managing Editor *Tessa Monina*
Proofreader *Nikky Twyman*
Art Director *Elaine Partington*
Designer *Malcolm Smythe*
Production *Sarah Rooney*

Line illustrations *Anthony Duke*